Musculoskeletal Ultrasound

Guest Editor

DIANA GAITINI, MD

ULTRASOUND CLINICS

www.ultrasound.theclinics.com

Consulting Editor
VIKRAM DOGRA, MD

October 2012 • Volume 7 • Number 4

SAUNDERS an imprint of ELSEVIER, Inc.

W.B. SAUNDERS COMPANY
A Division of Elsevier Inc.

1600 John F. Kennedy Boulevard ● Suite 1800 ● Philadelphia, Pennsylvania 19103-2899

http://www.theclinics.com

ULTRASOUND CLINICS Volume 7, Number 4
October 2012 ISSN 1556-858X, ISBN-13: 978-1-4557-3947-9

Editor: Donald Mumford

Ultrasound Clinics (ISSN 1556-858X) is published quarterly by W.B. Saunders, 360 Park Avenue South, New York, NY 10010-1710. Months of publication are January, April, July, and October. Business and editorial offices: 1600 John F. Kennedy Boulevard, Suite 1800, Philadelphia, Pennsylvania 19103-2899. Accounting and circulation offices: 6277 Sea Harbor Drive, Orlando, FL 32887-4800. Periodicals postage paid at New York, NY, and additional mailing offices. Subscription prices are $243 per year for (US individuals), $297 per year for (US institutions), $139 per year for (US students and residents), $273 per year for (Canadian individuals), $332 per year for (Canadian institutions), $291 per year for (international individuals), $332 per year for (international institutions), and $139 per year for (Canadian and foreign students/residents). To receive student/resident rate, orders must be accompanied by name of affiliated institution, date of term, and the signature of program/residency coordinator on institution letterhead. Orders will be billed at individual rate until proof of status is received. Foreign air speed delivery is included in all Clinics subscription prices. All prices are subject to change without notice. **POSTMASTER:** Send address changes to *Ultrasound Clinics,* Elsevier Health Sciences Division, Subscription Customer Service, 3251 Riverport Lane, Maryland Heights, MO 63043. **Customer Service (orders, claims, online, change of address): Telephone: 1-800-654-2452 (U.S. and Canada); 314-447-8871 (outside U.S. and Canada). Fax: 314-447-8029. E-mail: journalscustomerservice-usa@elsevier.com (for print support); journalsonlinesupport-usa@elsevier.com (for online support).**

Reprints: For copies of 100 or more, of articles in this publication, please contact the Commercial Reprints Department, Elsevier Inc., 360 Park Avenue South, New York, NY 10010-1710. Tel.: (+1) 212-633-3812; Fax: (+1) 212-462-1935; E-mail: reprints@elsevier.com.

Printed and bound by CPI Group (UK) Ltd, Croydon, CR0 4YY

Transferred to digital print 2012

Contributors

CONSULTING EDITOR

VIKRAM DOGRA, MD
Professor of Radiology, Urology, and
Biomedical Engineering, Director of Ultrasound
and Associate Chair for Education and
Research, Department of Imaging Sciences,
University of Rochester School of Medicine
and Dentistry, Rochester, New York

GUEST EDITOR

DIANA GAITINI, MD
Clinical Assistant Professor, Director, Unit of
Ultrasound, Department of Medical Imaging,
Rambam Health Care Center, Ruth and Bruce
Rappaport Faculty of Medicine, ITT- Israel
Institute of Technology, Haifa, Israel

AUTHORS

KIL-HO CHO, MD, PhD
Department of Diagnostic Radiology,
Yeungnam University Hospital, School
of Medicine, Yeungnam University, Daegu,
Korea

JOSEPH G. CRAIG, MB ChB
Staff Radiologist, Department of Radiology,
Henry Ford Hospital; Associate Clinical
Professor of Radiology, Wayne State
University Medical School, Detroit,
Michigan

NIRVIKAR DAHIYA, MD
Assistant Professor, Director-Ultrasound,
Section of Abdominal Imaging, Mallinckrodt
Institute of Radiology, Washington University
School of Medicine, St Louis, Missouri

TOBIAS DE ZORDO, MD
Department of Radiology, Medical University
Innsbruck, Tyrol, Austria

DAVID FESSELL, MD
Associate Professor of Radiology, University of
Michigan Medical School, Ann Arbor, Michigan

DIANA GAITINI, MD
Clinical Assistant Professor, Director, Unit of
Ultrasound, Department of Medical Imaging,
Rambam Health Care Center, Ruth and Bruce
Rappaport Faculty of Medicine, ITT- Israel
Institute of Technology, Haifa, Israel

JENN NEE KHOO, MB, BCh, BAO, FRCR (UK)
Department of Radiology, Changi General
Hospital, Singapore, Republic of Singapore

HOWARD PINCHCOFSKY, MD
Department of Diagnostic Radiology, Staff
Radiologist, Union Hospital of Cecil County,
Elkton, Maryland

CESARE ROMAGNOLI, MD, FRCPC
Department of Medical Imaging, Robarts
Research Institute, University of Western
Ontario, London, Ontario, Canada

RALF G. THIELE, MD
Assistant Professor of Medicine, Department of Medicine, Allergy/Immunology & Rheumatology Division, University of Rochester School of Medicine and Dentistry, Rochester, New York

IAN YU YAN TSOU, MBBS, FRCR (UK), MMed Imaging (Sydney)
Department of Diagnostic Radiology, Mount Elizabeth Hospital, Singapore, Republic of Singapore

GERVAIS KHIN-LIN WANSAICHEONG, MBBS, FRCR, MMed (Diagnostic Radiology)
Clinical Senior Lecturer, Yong Loo Lin School of Medicine, National University of Singapore, Singapore, Singapore

XIMENA WORTSMAN, MD
Departments of Radiology Dermatology, Clinica Servet, Faculty of Medicine, University of Chile, Santiago, Chile

Contents

precisely why ultrasound has an advantage over other imaging modalities. The higher spatial resolution and ability to perform dynamic maneuvers enables accurate diagnosis of many diseases affecting the region. Although history and physical examination remain the basis for the initial evaluation, ultrasound helps in excluding a more significant condition. This article describes the anatomy and pathology of commonly encountered lesions and provides a knowledge basis for evaluation of the ankle and foot.

There is a wide and growing spectrum of applications of sonography in the dermatologic field. Here, common causes of cutaneous and ungual lumps and bumps are reviewed, considering the technical requirements, and clinical and anatomic concepts. The usage of sonography in dermatology has gone beyond the experimental phase to become potentially an imaging technique in daily practice that provides anatomic and functional information otherwise unavailable to the clinical examination.

Ultrasonography has become a major imaging modality for rheumatologic indications. Advantages include detailed soft tissue visualization, if high frequency transducers are used for superficial structures such as small joints of hands and feet. Color or power Doppler ultrasonography can help identify inflamed tissues. Serial imaging provides information about disease status and helps monitor a treatment response. Ultrasound guidance of procedures in rheumatology leads to higher accuracy and better outcomes. Training specifically for rheumatologic indications is offered by the European League against Rheumatism and the American College of Rheumatology. Certification of proficiency can be obtained through the American College of Rheumatology.

Videos of ultrasound application to cyst injection; fragmentation and aspiration of calcific tendinosis; aspiration of masses; and foreign body removal accompany this article.

A wide variability of ultrasound-guided procedures are available and allow minimal invasive treatment of musculoskeletal disorders. This article describes general aspects of ultrasound-guided procedures in the musculoskeletal system. Also discussed are different interventional techniques, such as aspiration, injection, biopsy of soft tissue masses, aspiration and lavage of calcific tendinitis, and foreign body extraction. Finally, best approaches for single joints and tendons are delineated.

ULTRASOUND CLINICS

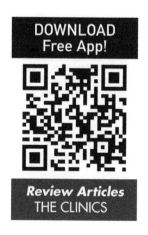

GOAL STATEMENT

The goal of the *Ultrasound Clinics* is to keep practicing radiologists and radiology residents up to date with current clinical practice in ultrasound by providing timely articles reviewing the state of the art in patient care.

ACCREDITATION

The *Ultrasound Clinics* is planned and implemented in accordance with the Essential Areas and Policies of the Accreditation Council for Continuing Medical Education (ACCME) through the joint sponsorship of the University of Virginia School of Medicine and Elsevier. The University of Virginia School of Medicine is accredited by the ACCME to provide continuing medical education for physicians.

The University of Virginia School of Medicine designates this enduring material activity for a maximum of 15 *AMA PRA Category 1 Credit*(s)™ for each issue, 60 credits per year. Physicians should claim only the credit commensurate with the extent of their participation in the activity.

The American Medical Association has determined that physicians not licensed in the US who participate in this CME enduring material activity are eligible for a maximum of 15 *AMA PRA Category 1 Credit*(s)™ for each issue, 60 credits per year.

Credit can be earned by reading the text material, taking the CME examination online at http://www.theclinics.com/home/cme, and completing the evaluation. After taking the test, you will be required to review any and all incorrect answers. Following completion of the test and evaluation, your credit will be awarded and you may print your certificate.

FACULTY DISCLOSURE/CONFLICT OF INTEREST

The University of Virginia School of Medicine, as an ACCME accredited provider, endorses and strives to comply with the Accreditation Council for Continuing Medical Education (ACCME) Standards of Commercial Support, Commonwealth of Virginia statutes, University of Virginia policies and procedures, and associated federal and private regulations and guidelines on the need for disclosure and monitoring of proprietary and financial interests that may affect the scientific integrity and balance of content delivered in continuing medical education activities under our auspices.

The University of Virginia School of Medicine requires that all CME activities accredited through this institution be developed independently and be scientifically rigorous, balanced and objective in the presentation/discussion of its content, theories and practices.

All authors/editors participating in an accredited CME activity are expected to disclose to the readers relevant financial relationships with commercial entities occurring within the past 12 months (such as grants or research support, employee, consultant, stock holder, member of speakers bureau, etc.). The University of Virginia School of Medicine will employ appropriate mechanisms to resolve potential conflicts of interest to maintain the standards of fair and balanced education to the reader. Questions about specific strategies can be directed to the Office of Continuing Medical Education, University of Virginia School of Medicine, Charlottesville, Virginia.

The faculty and staff of the University of Virginia Office of Continuing Medical Education have no financial affiliations to disclose.

The authors/editors listed below have identified no professional or financial affiliations for themselves or their spouse/partner:
Kil-Ho Cho, MD, PhD; Joseph G. Craig, MB ChB; Nirvikar Dahiya, MD; David Fessell, MD; Diana Gaitini, MD (Guest Editor); Jenn Nee Khoo, MB, BCh, BAO, FRCR; Donald Mumford, (Acquisitions Editor); Howard Pinchcofsky, MD; Cesare Romagnoli, MD, FRCPC; Ian Yu Yan Tsou, MBBS, FRCR, MMed Imaging; Gervais Khin-Lin Wansaicheong, MBBS, FRCR, Mmed; Ximena Wortsman, MD; and Tobias De Zordo, MD.

The authors/editors listed below have identified the following professional or financial affiliations for themselves or their spouse/partner:
Matthew J. Bassignani, MD (Test Author) is on the Advisory Board/Committee for Nuance and Fuji Medical Systems.
Vikram S. Dogra, MD (Consulting Editor) is the Editor of the Journal of Clinicl Imaging Science.
Ralf G. Thiele, MD is on the Speakers' Bureau for Abbott and Amgen, and receives equipment support from SonoSite.

Disclosure of Discussion of Non-FDA Approved Uses for Pharmaceutical Products and/or Medical Devices.
The University of Virginia School of Medicine, as an ACCME provider, requires that all faculty presenters identify and disclose any off-label uses for pharmaceutical and medical device products. The University of Virginia School of Medicine recommends that each physician fully review all the available data on new products or procedures prior to clinical use.

TO ENROLL

To enroll in the Ultrasound Clinics Continuing Medical Education program, call customer service at 1-800-654-2452 or visit us online at www.theclinics.com/home/cme. The CME program is available to subscribers for an additional fee of $196.00.

Preface
Musculoskeletal Ultrasound

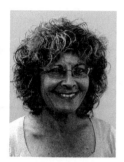

Diana Gaitini, MD
Guest Editor

As we prepare this *Ultrasound Clinics* issue on Musculoskeletal Ultrasound, the 2012 Olympic Games in London are running and the world is watching with enthusiasm and admiration. In the background, collectively, millions of hours of training are evident. Sports are a dangerous activity, leading in many cases to injuries of every kind. Not long ago there was no place for ultrasound in the diagnostic battery. Since then, the development of high-resolution multifrequency linear transducers together with the knowledge and skills of ultrasound operators have brought this modality into wide use, making it the first imaging choice for the diagnosis of musculoskeletal pathologies. In many respects, there is no competition with any other modality. The ability to produce images in real-time and during dynamic maneuvers demonstrates flow even at extremely low velocities and the exquisite spatial resolution, not achieved by any other imaging modality, has made ultrasound a unique tool for musculoskeletal diagnoses. Not to mention the low cost, lack of ionizing radiation, iodinated contrast media or gadolinium, wide availability, portability, patient comfort, and fastness. The development of minimally invasive diagnostic procedures by biopsying lesions under imaging guidance placed ultrasound as the first modality to guide biopsies and, furthermore, to perform local treatments, like anesthetic and steroid injections, radiofrequency, breaking up of calcifications, blood injection for tears treatment, and more, with the ability to follow through a needle track over the whole way, placing the tip of the needle in the exact point, and avoiding vital structures like vessels or nerves. Tendons, ligaments, nerves, vessels, muscles, fat, and even skin can be precisely analyzed and any pathological finding diagnosed. But, as always in life, nothing is perfect, and there is in this modality an important drawback, which is its operator-dependence. More than in any other modality, where images are automatically performed, ultrasound depends on the skill of the operator to be done correctly and any image is the product of their knowledge of anatomy and pathology of the area being examined, together with the knowledge of the physical and technical principles of ultrasound. Selection of frequency and type of transducer, gain, depth, focus, penetration range, use of panoramic view, harmonics, color/spectral Doppler, just to mention a few, are tasks of the operator. This was the goal in conceiving this issue of *Ultrasound Clinics*: to aid in achieving the required knowledge and skills for a proper performance of musculoskeletal ultrasound. Thanks to the efforts of people experienced in this field writing the articles and presenting the pictures and videos, we produced a practical and friendly issue, with the hope of adding to the development of this unique field.

Ultrasound Clin 7 (2012) ix–x
http://dx.doi.org/10.1016/j.cult.2012.08.018
1556-858X/12/$ – see front matter

I am deeply thankful to Professor Vikram Dogra, outstanding ultrasound professional, teacher, and mentor, for giving me the opportunity of editing this issue. I thank Donald Mumford, Elsevier editor, for his efforts in getting it done on time. Above all, I am very grateful to all the authors who dedicated time and efforts in making it possible. No doubt, the lectors will be the judges, and we do hope that they will find it useful to keep at hand and valuable in their day-to-day practice.

Diana Gaitini, MD
Ruth and Bruce Rappaport Faculty of Medicine
ITT—Israel Institute of Technology
Unit of Ultrasound
Department of Medical Imaging
Rambam Health Care Center
8 Ha'aliya, POB 9602
Haifa, Israel 31096

E-mail address:
d_gaitini@rambam.health.gov.il

The Shoulder
Rotator Cuff Pathology and Beyond

Diana Gaitini, MD[a],*, Nirvikar Dahiya, MD[b]

KEYWORDS

- Shoulder ultrasonography • Shoulder anatomy • Rotator cuff tear • Impingement syndrome
- Bursitis

KEY POINTS

- A complete systematic ultrasound examination of the shoulder is essential to obtain a correct diagnosis, as the clinical presentation is fairly accurate.
- Proper operator skills and high-resolution transducers are required.
- Patient positioning must be adequate for every stage of rotator cuff evaluation.
- Anisotropy artifact must be avoided by correct transducer positioning, perpendicular to the tendon.
- Static imaging of the rotator cuff must be supplemented by a dynamic examination.
- Postoperative rotator cuff has a significantly variable appearance than a normal cuff and artifacts from suture material and anchors should not be construed as tears.

 Videos of dynamic maneuvers performances accompany this article.

Shoulder ultrasound (US) has become one of the most common examinations performed in musculoskeletal imaging. Modern US equipment with high-frequency transducers allows for high-quality imaging, with even higher resolution capacities than magnetic resonance imaging (MRI).[1] The ability to visualize structures in real time in both static and dynamic states, and evaluate vascularity without injecting contrast agents, offers compelling advantages over MRI. The main drawback of US is its operator-dependence, where examination accuracy varies with the operator's skill and experience.[2] A complete systematic examination is essential to obtain a high-level musculoskeletal sonograph that competes with MRI.[3] A strict examination protocol should be followed. We describe the scanning technique and normal anatomy as the first steps toward performing an effective shoulder US evaluation.

SCANNING TECHNIQUE AND NORMAL ANATOMY

A 12-MHz to 15-MHz linear array transducer for an average-sized patient will provide enough penetration to achieve excellent resolution. A 9-MHz frequency is needed in a larger patient to achieve deeper penetration, obviously at the expense of resolution.[4–6] The sequential steps for US evaluation of the shoulder are presented in **Box 1**.

Long Head of the Biceps Brachii Tendon

The patient is seated on a rolling stool facing the operator, the arm in neutral or slight internal rotation, palm-up hand on the thigh. The transducer is placed in the axial plane over the anterior humeral head (**Fig. 1A**). The lesser and greater tuberosities are the bony landmarks to identify the bicipital groove. The long head of the biceps brachii tendon

The authors have nothing to disclose.
[a] Unit of Ultrasound, Department of Medical Imaging, Rambam Health Care Center, Ruth and Bruce Rappaport Faculty of Medicine, ITT- Israel Institute of Technology, 8 Ha'aliya, POB 9602, Haifa 31096, Israel; [b] Clinical Ultrasound, Section of Abdominal Imaging, Mallinckrodt Institute of Radiology, Washington University School of Medicine, 510 South Kingshighway Boulevard, Campus Box 8131, St Louis, MO 63110, USA
* Corresponding author. Unit of Ultrasound, Department of Medical Imaging, Rambam Health Care Center, 8 Ha'aliya, POB 9602, Haifa 31096, Israel.
E-mail address: d_gaitini@rambam.health.gov.il

is seen in short axis within the bicipital groove as a rounded hyperechogenic structure (**Fig. 1B**). Anisotropy, an artifact that makes the tendon appear hypoechoic (**Fig. 1C**), may be avoided by a slight tilting of the probe so it is superiorly angled and perpendicular to the tendon. The biceps tendon is followed from the proximal humeral head distally to the level of the insertion of the pectoralis major on the lateral aspect of the bicipital groove. The transducer is then turned 90°, placing it along the humeral shaft for a longitudinal view of the biceps tendon (**Fig. 1D**). The normal fibrillar hyperechoic tendon structure is seen (**Fig. 1E**).

The tendon is followed from the intra-articular portion in the rotator interval, which is a space between the subscapularis and the supraspinatus tendon, to the distal musculo-tendinous junction. A minimal amount of fluid posterior to the tendon is considered physiologic.

Subscapularis Tendon

The patient is asked to externally rotate the shoulder by forearm abduction of the flexed arm. The transducer is placed in a transverse plane medial to the bicipital groove to obtain a longitudinal view of the subscapularis tendon (**Fig. 2A**). The tendon is seen as a fibrillar hyperechoic structure (**Fig. 2B**). The transducer is then rotated 90° to obtain an axial view of the tendon (**Fig. 2C**). On short view, a series of hypoechoic clefts, related to muscle fibers interposed with the hyperechogenic tendon fibers are seen (**Fig. 2D**).

Supraspinatus Tendon and Subacromial Subdeltoid Bursa

The patient is asked to place the dorsum of the hand on the opposite lower back (Crass position). A modified Crass or Middleton position is recommended to lower patient discomfort, consisting of the palm of the hand placed on the ipsilateral waist, the elbow

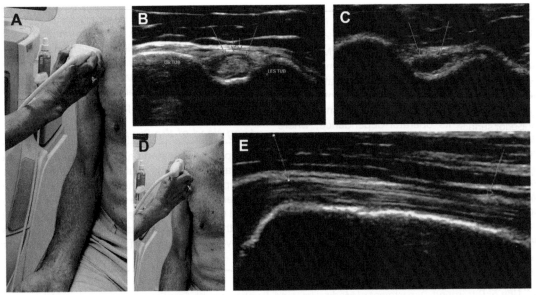

Fig. 1. Long head of the biceps brachii tendon. (*A*) Axial scan. The patient is facing the operator, palm-up hand on the thigh. The transducer is placed perpendicular to the tendon in the axial plane. (*B*) Axial view. The biceps tendon is seen as a rounded fibrillar hyperechogenic structure (*long arrows*) inside the concave bicipital groove between the lesser (LES TUB) and greater (GR TUB) tuberosities. Above the biceps tendon, the transverse humeral ligament is seen (*short arrows*). (*C*) Anisotropy artifact. The tendon appears artifactually hypoechoic (*arrows*) when the transducer is not perpendicular to it. (*D*) Longitudinal scan. The transducer is placed parallel to the tendon in the sagittal plane. (*E*) The tendon is seen as a fine fibrillar hyperechoic structure from the intra-articular area to the musculotendinous junction (*arrows*).

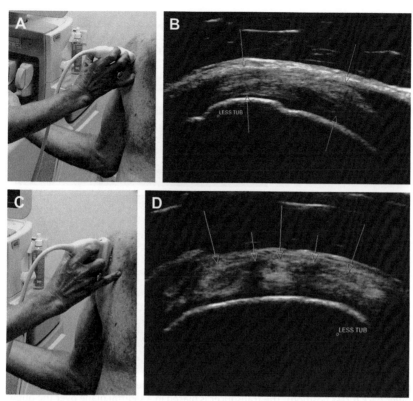

Fig. 2. Subscapularis tendon. (*A*) The patient's shoulder is externally rotated by abduction of the forearm. The transducer is placed in an axial plane for a long view of the tendon. (*B*) Long view. The tendon is seen as an echogenic band (*arrows*) over the humeral head inserting on the lesser tuberosity (LESS TUB). (*C*) The transducer is placed in a sagittal plane for a short view of the tendon. (*D*) Short view. The hyperechogenic tendon (*long arrows*) intercalating with hypoechogenic muscle fibers (*short arrows*) is seen, inserting in the lesser tuberosity (LESS TUB).

pointing posteriorly. The transducer is placed in a sagittal plane over the humeral head laterally to the bicipital groove (**Fig. 3**A). The fibrillar hyperechogenic tendon is seen in the long view with a convex superior surface, underneath the echogenic subcromial subdeltoid bursa and the hypoechogenic deltoid muscle (**Fig. 3**B). Below the tendon, the hyperechoic humeral head is visible, covered by the hypoechoic hyaline articular cartilage. The transducer is then turned 90° to scan the supraspinatus tendon in the short axis (**Fig. 3**C). In short view, the fibrillar hyperechoic tendon should be followed from the hyperechogenic biceps tendon anteriorly to the infraspinatus tendon posteriorly, the last represented by several thin hypoechoic lines owing to anisotropy. The collapsed subacromial subdeltoid bursa is seen above the supraspinatus tendon as a hyperechoic line, sometimes with a minimal amount of fluid inside (**Fig. 3**D).

Infraspinatus and Teres Minor Tendons

The infraspinatus and teres minor tendons are examined from the posterior shoulder. The patient is asked to rotate so his or her back is facing the operator, placing the ipsilateral hand in neutral position or over the opposite shoulder (**Fig. 4**A). The transducer is placed in the infraspinatus fossa, just below the scapular spine. A longitudinal view of the infraspinatus tendon is obtained by placing the transducer in a slightly oblique axial plane. The infraspinatus tendon is seen as a thick, hyperechogenic beak-shaped structure extending over the posterior humeral head and under the deltoid muscle (**Fig. 4**B). The transducer is then rotated 90° (**Fig. 4**C). The large infraspinatus tendon in short axis and the small and more superficial teres minor tendon are seen (**Fig. 4**D). Both tendons insert in the posterior aspect of the greater tuberosity.

Glenohumeral Joint and Spinoglenoid Notch

The transducer is displaced medially in an axial plane (**Fig. 5**A). The humeral head cortex and the glenoid tuberosity conforming the glenohumeral joint are seen. A triangular hyperechogenic structure in-between represents the posterior cartilage labrum (**Fig. 5**B). The transducer is then moved

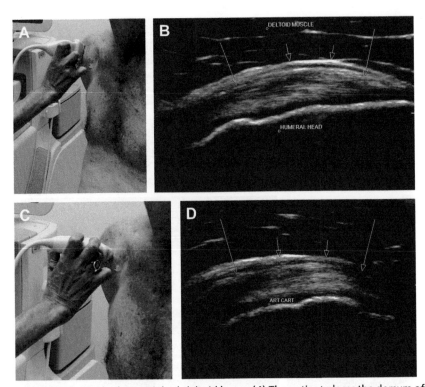

Fig. 3. Supraspinatus tendon and subacromial subdeltoid bursa. (*A*) The patient places the dorsum of the hand on the opposite lower back (Crass position). The transducer is placed in a sagittal plane over the humeral head, laterally to the bicipital groove. (*B*) Long view. The fibrillar medium level echogenic tendon is seen (*long arrows*) overlying the hypoechogenic articular cartilage on the humeral head (HUMERAL HEAD) and underneath the echogenic subcromial subdeltoid bursa (*short arrows*) and the deltoid muscle (DELTOID MUSCLE). (*C*) The transducer is rotated to the axial plane. (*D*) Short view. The supraspinatus tendon (*long arrows*) extends laterally from the intra-articular portion of the biceps longus, underneath the hyperechoic subacromial subdeltoid bursa (*short arrows*) and above the articular cartilage (ART CART).

slightly medially to show the spinoglenoid notch (**Fig. 5**C). The notch appears as a concave echogenic bone structure (**Fig. 5**D). The suprascapular nerve and vessels run inside the notch; the artery may be seen on color Doppler.

Acromioclavicular Joint

The patient is then positioned in front of the examiner and the hand is returned to the lap, palm up. The transducer is placed over the acromion and distal clavicle in a coronal plane to scan the acromioclavicular joint (**Fig. 6**A). The hyperechogenic bone contours of the acromion and the distal clavicle and the interposed hypoechoic wedge-shaped fibrocartilagenous tissue are seen (**Fig. 6**B).

Dynamic Maneuvers

Dynamic maneuvers are performed to rule out subacromial impingement. The transducer is placed over the acromial edge and the supraspinatus tendon and subacromial subdeltoid bursa are identified. The patient is asked to abduct the arm in

internal rotation by raising the elbow laterally (**Fig. 7**A), and then to extend the arm anteriorly with the hand in pronation (**Fig. 7**B). The supraspinatus tendon and subacromial subdeltoid bursa are seen gliding underneath the acromion while performing the dynamic maneuvers (**Fig. 7**C) (videos 1 and 2).

ROTATOR CUFF PATHOLOGY

Rotator cuff disease is a common source of pain in patients older than 40 years, the frequency increasing with age.[7]

Rotator Cuff Tendinopathy or Tendinosis

Rotator cuff tendinopathy or tendinosis primarily affects the supraspinatus tendon, as a consequence of anterosuperior subacromial impingement. The tendon appears swollen and has a heterogeneous echotexture (**Fig. 8**). Supraspinatus tendinosis is often associated with thickening of the subacromial subdeltoid bursa and a small reactive bursal effusion.

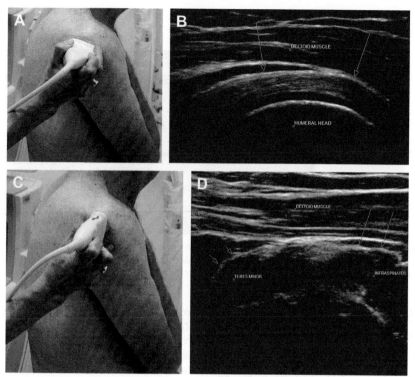

Fig. 4. Infraspinatus and teres minor tendons. (*A*) The patient's back is facing the operator, the hand placed over the opposite shoulder. The transducer is placed on the infraspinatus fossa in a slightly oblique axial plane. (*B*) Long view. The infraspinatus tendon (*arrows*) is seen extending over the posterior humeral head (HUMERAL HEAD) and under the deltoid muscle (DELTOID MUSCLE). (*C*) The transducer is rotated to a perpendicular plane. (*D*) Short view. The large infraspinatus tendon (*long arrows*) and the small teres minor tendon (*short arrows*) are seen. Infraspinatus muscle (INFRASPINATUS) and teres minor muscle (TERES MINOR).

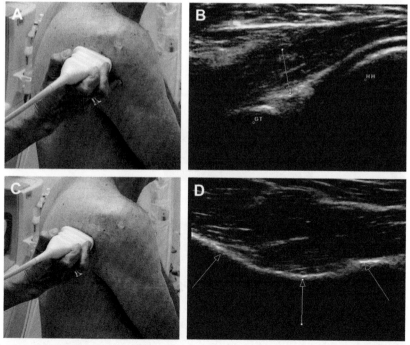

Fig. 5. Glenohumeral joint and spinoglenoid notch. (*A*) Patient positioning is unchanged, the transducer is placed slightly lower and medially in an axial plane. (*B*) Glenohumeral joint and posterior labrum. The humeral head cortex (HH), the glenoid tuberosity (GT), and the triangular glenoid posterior cartilage labrum (*arrow*) are seen. (*C*) Spinoglenoid notch. The transducer is moved slightly medially. (*D*) The spinoglenoid notch appears as a concave echogenic bone structure (*long arrows*).

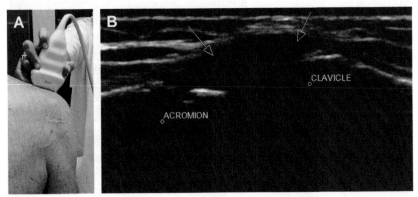

Fig. 6. Acromioclavicular joint. (*A*) The transducer is placed over the acromion in a coronal plane. (*B*) The acromial (ACROMION) and clavicular (CLAVICLE) bone articular surfaces and the interposed hypoechoic wedge-shaped fibrocartilagenous disk (*arrows*) are seen.

Rotator Cuff Tears

Tears are a common cause of shoulder pain. US offers comparable accuracy to MRI for the diagnosis of tendon tears, with more than 90% sensitivity and specificity when performed by an experienced examiner with high-end equipment.[7,8] The different types of rotator cuff tears are summarized in **Box 2**. *Partial-thickness tears* are seen as a hypoechoic or anechoic area in the tendon, detected in both longitudinal and axial planes. According to the localization, partial tears are

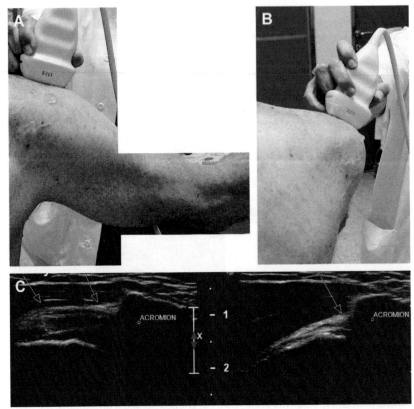

Fig. 7. Dynamic maneuvers. (*A*) The transducer is placed over the anterior end of the acromion and the patient is asked to raise the arm. (*B*) The patient is asked to extend the arm forward. (*C*) The normal supraspinatus tendon and subacromial subdeltoid bursa are seen at rest (*left plot, arrows*) and sliding to hide under the acromion (ACROMION) during dynamic maneuvers (*right plot, arrow*) (videos 1 and 2).

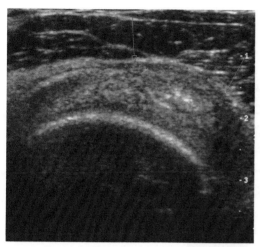

Fig. 8. Rotator cuff tendinopathy or tendinosis. A thickened supraspinatus tendon with a heterogeneous echotexture is seen (*arrows*).

classified into bursal surface, articular surface, and intrasubstance tears. Bursal surface tears are less common but better delineated by fluid entering the cleft (**Fig. 9**A). Tears involving the tendon articular surface are commoner, often associated with irregularities of the underlying cortical bone. The hypoechogenic articular cartilage is clearly seen owing to the interface with the anechoic tear (**Fig. 9**B). Intrasubstance tears are seen as a cleft confined to the tendon width, making it difficult to differentiate from focal tendinosis (**Fig. 9**C). *Full-thickness tears* extend through the tendon from the bursal to the articular surface, connecting the subdeltoid bursa with the articular surface (**Fig. 10**A). Tears most frequently affect the anterior third of the supraspinatus tendon, at the level of the so-called "critical zone," a relatively hypovascular area placed about 1 cm medially to the tendon attachment on the greater tuberosity (**Fig. 10**B). Useful indirect signs of full-thickness tears are an upper concavity at the level of the tear owing to

---

Box 2
Types of rotator cuff tears

1. Partial-thickness tears

   a. Bursal surface tendon tear

   b. Articular surface tendon tear

   c. Intrasubstance tear

2. Full-thickness tears

   a. Focal full-thickness tendon tear

   b. Complete full-thickness full-width tendon tear

   c. Massive rotator cuff tendon tear

---

focal bursal herniation, and a clear visualization of the articular cartilage beneath it, by the interface between the hypoechogenic cartilage and the anechoic fluid into the tear, which is the "uncovered or cartilage interface sign." *Complete tears* refer to full-thickness tears involving the full width of the tendon, which retracts beneath the acromion, leaving the humeral head and greater tuberosity without rotator cuff covering (**Fig. 10**C). Size and location of the tear and degree of retraction of the torn tendon should be reported.[7] *Massive tears* affect the whole rotator cuff, from a complete tear of the supraspinatus tendon extending anteriorly to the subscapularis and posteriorly to the infraspinatus (**Fig. 10**D).

Calcifying Tendinitis

Calcifying tendinitis refers to calcium deposition in the tendons, predominantly hydroxyapatite, most commonly in the supraspinatus tendon. Three types of tendon calcifications have been described.[1] Type I calcifications are seen as hyperechoic rounded or linear foci, with well-defined acoustic shadow (**Fig. 11**A), corresponding to the formative phase of the calcium deposit. Types II and III correspond to the resorptive phase, in which the deposits are nearly liquid. Type II calcifications are hyperechoic foci with a faint posterior shadow (**Fig. 11**B). In Type III, the acoustic shadow is absent. Calcific deposits, especially Types II and III, may migrate to a subbursal position and even penetrate the bursa, which is shown with thickened walls and filled with hyperechoic fluid (**Fig. 11**C).

Impingement Syndrome

Impingement is related to supraspinatus tendon damage caused by chronic contact of the tendon with the coracoacromial arch. The arch is formed by the anterior part of the acromion, the acromioclavicular joint, the coracoacromial ligament, and the tip of the coracoid. It is considered the main source of tendon tears.[9] A restrictive subacromial space, owing to congenital or acquired bone morphology or a thickened supraspinatus tendon or subacromial bursa, prevent normal tendon movement in the subacromial space on abduction and elevation of the arm, leading to tendon impingement (**Fig. 12**).

SHOULDER PATHOLOGY BEYOND THE ROTATOR CUFF
Biceps Tendon Pathology

Fluid may be seen surrounding the biceps tendon and can be a normal finding. When the amount of fluid is large and the tendon is thick with irregular

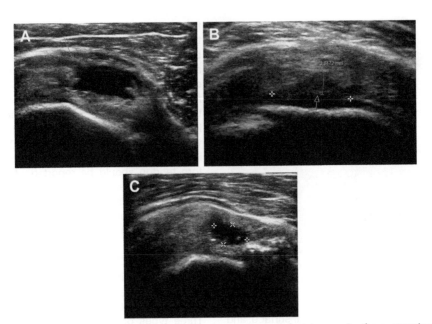

Fig. 9. Partial-thickness tears. (*A*) Bursal surface tear. An anechoic defect is seen in the supraspinatus tendon reaching the subdeltoid bursa (*arrows*). (*B*) Articular surface tear. The underneath hypoechogenic articular cartilage is well delineated (*arrow*) owing to the interface with the anechoic tear (*cursors*). (*C*) Intrasubstance tear. A sonolucent defect into the supraspinatus tendon width is seen (*cursors*).

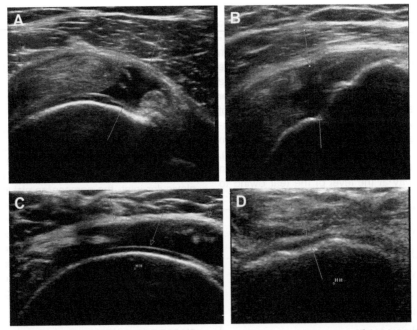

Fig. 10. Full-thickness and complete tears. (*A*) Short axis. Full-thickness tendon tear without retraction. A sonolucent tendon defect is seen involving the whole tendon thickness (*arrows*). (*B*) Long axis. The tear is seen at the level of the "critical zone." (*C*) Complete full-thickness tear with tendon retraction. The tear involves the full width of the tendon revealing the whole articular cartilage (*large arrow*) and the above-placed subdeltoid bursa (*short arrows*). HH, humeral head. (*D*) Massive tear. The whole rotator cuff is involved. The subdeltoid bursa (*short arrow*) is seen in contact with the articular cartilage (*long arrow*). No rotator cuff covering is seen over the humeral head (HH).

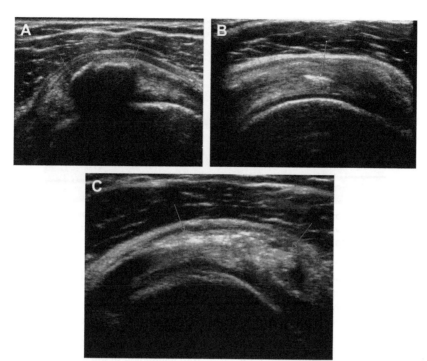

Fig. 11. Calcifying tendinitis. (*A*) Type I calcification. Large focal calcifications with a clear posterior acoustic shadow are seen in the supraspinatus tendon (*arrows*). (*B*) Type II calcification. A hyperechogenic foci with a faint posterior acoustic shadow (*arrow*) is seen. (*C*) Type III calcifications. Calcified deposits in the tendon without acoustic shadowing extruding into the bursa and hyperechogenic fluid filling the bursa are seen (*arrows*).

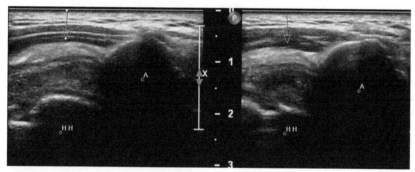

Fig. 12. Impingement syndrome. Left plot: static image of the tendon and bursa (*arrow*) above the humeral head (HH) and below the acromiocoracoid arch (A). Right plot: on dynamic maneuvers, the supraspinatus tendon and the subacromial subdeltoid bursa (*arrow*) are entrapped in the narrow corridor between the humeral head (HH) and the acromiocoracoid arch (A).

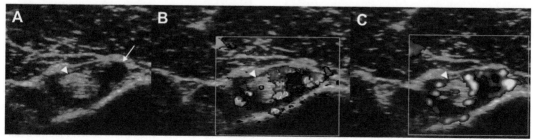

Fig. 13. Biceps tenosynovitis. Gray scale (*A*), color Doppler (*B*), and power Doppler (*C*) images taken in a transverse plane at the bicipital groove. Biceps tendon (*arrowhead*) surrounded by fluid within the tendon sheath (*arrow*) with profuse increase in vascularity, seen on color (*B*) and power (*C*) Doppler.

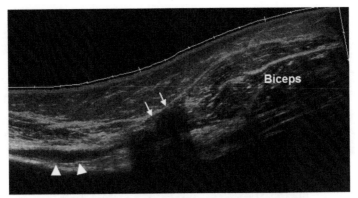

Fig. 14. Ruptured biceps tendon. Extended field of view in a longitudinal plane shows a ruptured biceps tendon with retracted distal edge toward the biceps muscle (Biceps). Refractive shadowing from the retracted tendon (*arrows*) and an empty bicipital groove (*arrowheads*) are seen.

borders, it raises the possibility of tendinitis.[10] Recent literature prefers to use the term "tendinosis" to describe chronically inflamed tendons. Color Doppler helps in looking for increased vascularity within the tendon and the sheath in acute presentation. Increased vascularity is associated with tenosynovitis (**Fig. 13**). Increased fluid around the biceps tendon may also indicate the presence of a rotator cuff tear, especially if fluid is also seen in the subdeltoid bursa.[11]

Nonvisualization of the tendon within the grove should raise the possibility of a ruptured tendon that may have retracted inferiorly. Extended field of view can be used to show the retracted end of the tendon and the empty groove (**Fig. 14**). Sometimes the tendon may be dislocated medially (**Fig. 15**) and if the bicipital groove is empty, the search for biceps tendon should extend medial to the lesser tuberosity. A medially dislocated tendon may be associated with a coexisting subscapularis tendon tear, because the subscapularis tendon contributes some fibers to the rotator

interval capsule that keeps the biceps tendon within the groove.[12]

Subacromial/Subdeltoid Bursitis

Subacromial/subdeltoid bursitis usually presents with thickening of the bursa with or without fluid.[13] Usually the bursa is thick and hypoechoic, although it may even be heterogeneous (**Fig. 16**). If there is difficulty in identifying the bursa confidently, dynamic evaluation by abducting the arm resolves the issue. This may be associated with impingement syndrome, as discussed previously.

Adhesive Capsulitis—Frozen Shoulder

The term "frozen shoulder" has been used historically to describe symptoms of a shoulder that shows limitation of movement. In strictest sense, adhesive capsulitis is a syndrome defined as an idiopathic painful restriction of the shoulder

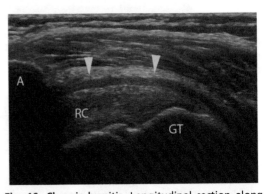

Fig. 16. Chronic bursitis. Longitudinal section along the posterior rotator cuff (RC) shows significant thickening of the subdeltoid bursa (*arrowheads*). Medially placed acromium (A) and lateral insertion of the rotator cuff at the greater tuberosity (GT) are visualized.

Fig. 15. Dislocated biceps tendon. Transverse section at the level of the subscapularis (Sub S) tendon shows a medially dislocated biceps tendon (*arrowhead*) overlying the lesser tuberosity (LT).

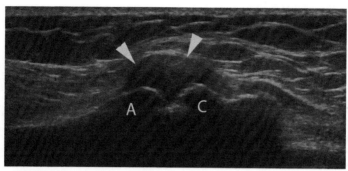

Fig. 17. Acromio-clavicular arthritis. Transverse section through the acromioclavicular joint shows hypertrophy of the joint capsule (*arrowheads*) with decreased joint space between the acromial (A) and the clavicular (C) ends of the joint.

movement with global restriction of the glenohumeral joint. It has been suggested to use the term "adhesive capsulitis" to refer to the primary idiopathic condition and the term "secondary adhesive capsulitis" to refer to conditions that are a result of other pathologic etiologies that may include adherent or obliterative bursitis.[14] The patient presents with a painful and restrictive shoulder joint. Systemic diseases like diabetes, hyperthyroidism, and rheumatoid arthritis may be associated with secondary adhesive capsulitis.[15,16] The main role of US is in identifying other causes of pain or restriction, such as rotator cuff tears, tenosynovitis, calcific tendinitis, and subdeltoid bursitis. Idiopathic adhesive capsulitis is a diagnosis of exclusion. US may demonstrate a hypoechoic soft mass and increased vascularity in the rotator interval and thickening of the coracohumeral ligament.[17,18]

Acromioclavicular Joint Pathologies

The ligaments that are responsible for the integrity of the acromioclavicular joint are the coracoacromial ligament, coracoclavicular ligament, and trapezoid

and conoid components attaching to the undersurface of the clavicle.[19] Hypertrophy of the overlying ligaments (**Fig. 17**), capsule, cysts, and bony erosions represent the spectrum of degenerative changes.[20] A cyst or ganglion projecting superiorly from the joint may be present in rotator cuff tears when fluid from the subdeltoid bursa extends through the joint also known as the "geyser" sign.[21]

Humeral Head Fractures

In the presence of history of trauma sometimes a subtle step off may be seen along the contour of the humeral head that may represent a small fracture (**Fig. 18**). There may be an associated hematoma in the soft tissue or even a coexistent rotator cuff tear. Cortical irregularity and bony erosions should not be mistaken for a fracture.[22]

POSTOPERATIVE SHOULDER

Although the term "postoperative shoulder" is all encompassing, we limit the description to the normal and abnormal appearances of a rotator cuff that has undergone surgical repair of

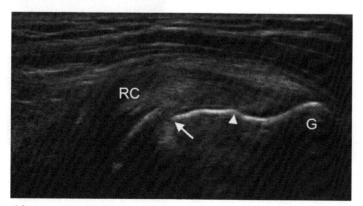

Fig. 18. Humeral head fracture. Longitudinal image through the posterior rotator cuff (RC) shows a step-off in the contour of the humeral head (*arrow*) representing the fracture. The arrowhead points out the lateral margin of the articular cartilage at the anatomic neck of the humerus. The rotator cuff inserts at the greater tuberosity (G).

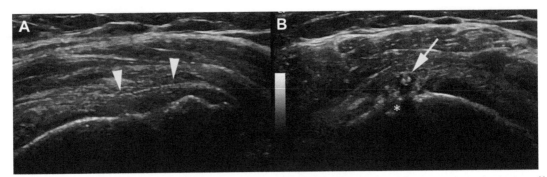

Fig. 19. Postoperative rotator cuff. Longitudinal (*A*) and transverse (*B*) images of the post repaired rotator cuff showing suture material (*arrowheads*) traversing the substance of the cuff and anchor screw (*arrow*) at the reimplantation trough (*asterisk*).

a tear. Large studies have not been done to assess the accuracy of US in detection of postoperative rotator cuff. Prickett and colleagues[23] evaluated 44 patients and reported a sensitivity, specificity, and accuracy of US for identifying rotator cuff integrity at 91%, 86%, and 89%, respectively.

Surgery of the rotator cuff can either be a simple debridement of granulation tissue at a partial-thickness tear, or a tendon-to-tendon or tendon-to-bone repair. Prior history is helpful in knowing details about the type of surgery performed. Types of rotator cuff repair constructs include transosseous repairs, single-row repairs, or double-row repairs. Transosseous repairs use open and mini-open techniques in which sutures are placed directly through transosseous tunnels for soft tissue fixation. Single-row repairs are done by placing the anchors in a linear fashion within the center of tuberosity footprint and double-row repairs include techniques that use a medial row of suture anchors at the articular cartilage margin of the anatomic neck with a second more lateral row of anchors at the edge of the rotator cuff footprint along the tuberosity.[24]

After a surgical repair for tear, the "normal" appearance of a repaired tendon is heterogeneous with curving echogenic lines traversing the substance of the cuff representing suture material. Stronger hyperechoic artifact in the cuff that shadows may represent anchor screws in the reimplantation trough (**Fig. 19**). The repaired tendon may appear thick or thin, and is not necessarily abnormal. A small amount of fluid within the tendon may even be normal. Rotator cuffs that are post repair are not watertight and communication between the glenohumeral joint and subacromial/subdeltoid bursa may be present. Most recurrent tears appear as complete absence of the cuff (**Fig. 20**). If the cuff has not retracted, a fluid-filled defect may be seen with some flimsy remnant tendon fibers or suture material within the defect (**Fig. 21**). Small recurrent tears are difficult to

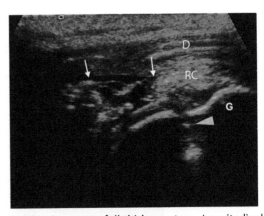

Fig. 20. Complete full-thickness recurrent tear. Longitudinal section of the rotator cuff. There is no cuff visible. The deltoid (D) muscle rests on the humerus (H). The arrowheads represent the empty reimplantation trough, possibly secondary to a displaced anchor. GT, greater tuberosity.

Fig. 21. Recurrent full-thickness tear. Longitudinal section of the rotator cuff (RC) shows a defect (*arrows*) within the cuff with flimsy linear echoes traversing the defect that may represent a combination of some remnant fibers and suture material. The arrowhead shows the site of the suture anchor. G, greater tuberosity; D, deltoid muscle.

> **What the referring physician should be aware of**
>
> - Painful arc syndrome is a clinical description of pain on arm abduction above shoulder height, or shoulder pain occurring at night, sometimes to the point of waking the patient.[27]
> - Pain is derived from the rotator cuff and the subacromial bursa passing beneath the coracoacromial arch.
> - Rotator cuff disease increases with age.
> - Supraspinatus tendonitis, rotator cuff tear, subacromial bursitis, subacromial impingement, and acromioclavicular joint inflammation or degenerative changes may be the source of pain.
> - Often, no signs or symptoms can reliably distinguish between the variety of pathologies.
> - Imaging using either US or MRI is the standard means by which a differential diagnosis may be reached.
> - The history and clinical examination are crucial in determining the need for subsequent imaging examination.
> - A radiograph of the shoulder in the presence of signs and symptoms of rotator cuff pathology would be indicated in a patient with a history of trauma to rule out fractures; in the elderly, to identify degenerative changes; and in patients with acute onset of severe unremitting shoulder pain, to rule out calcifying tendinitis or bursitis and bone tumors.

appreciate unless a prior baseline postoperative examination is available. There may be hypoechoic scar tissue in the subacromial/subdeltoid bursal space. Fluid within the subdeltoid bursal space and muscle atrophy may be present.[25,26]

SUPPLEMENTARY DATA

Videos related to this article can be found online at http://dx.doi.org/10.1016/j.cult.2012.08.005.

REFERENCES

1. Bianchi S, Martinoli C. Shoulder. In: Martinoli C, Bianchi S, editors. Ultrasound of the musculoskeletal system. Berlin and Heidelberg (Germany): Springer & Verlag; 2007. p. 189–331.
2. Le Corroler T, Cohen M, Aswad R, et al. Sonography of the painful shoulder: role of the operator's experience. Skeletal Radiol 2009;37:979–86.
3. Jamadar JA, Jacobson JA, Caoili EM, et al. Musculoskeletal sonography technique: focused versus comprehensive evaluation. Am J Roentgenol 2008; 190:5–9.
4. Jacobson JA. Shoulder US: anatomy, technique and scanning pitfalls. Radiology 2011;260:6–16.
5. Gaitini D, Militianu D, Nachtigal A, et al. Shoulder. In: Dogra V, Gaitini D, editors. Musculoskeletal ultrasound with MRI correlations. Stuttgart (Germany) & New York: Thieme Medical Publishers; 2010. p. 1–21.
6. Gaitini D. Shoulder ultrasonography: performance and common findings. J Clin Imaging Sci 2012;2:38.
7. Moosikasuwan JB, Miller TT, Burke BJ. Rotator cuff tears: clinical, radiographic and US findings. Radiographics 2005;25:1591–607.
8. Teefey SA, Rubin DA, Middleton WD, et al. Detection and quantification of rotator cuff tears: comparison of ultrasonography, magnetic resonance imaging and arthroscopic findings in seventy-one consecutive cases. J Bone Joint Surg Am 2004;86:708–16.
9. Bureau NJ, Beauchamp M, Cardinal E, et al. Dynamic sonography evaluation of shoulder impingement syndrome. Am J Roentgenol 2006;26:1045–65.
10. Farin PU. Sonography of the biceps tendon of the shoulder: normal and pathologic findings. J Clin Ultrasound 1996;24:309–16.
11. Teefey SA, Middleton WD, Yamaguchi K. Shoulder sonography: state of the art. Radiol Clin North Am 1999;37:767–85.
12. Symeonides PP. The significance of the subscapularis muscle in the pathogenesis of recurrent anterior dislocations of the shoulder. J Bone Joint Surg Br 1972;54:276–483.
13. Farin PU, Jaroma H, Harju A, et al. Shoulder impingement syndrome: sonographic evaluation. Radiology 1990;176:845–9.
14. Siegel LB, Cohen NJ, Gall EP. Adhesive capsulitis: a sticky issue. Am Fam Physician 1999;59: 1843–50.
15. Wohlgethan JR. Frozen shoulder in hyperthyroidism. Arthritis Rheum 1987;30:936–9.
16. Arkkila PE, Kantola IM, Viikari JS, et al. Shoulder capsulitis in type I and II diabetic patients. Ann Rheum Dis 1996;55:907–14.
17. Lee JC, Sykes C, Saifuddin A, et al. Adhesive capsulitis: sonographic changes in the rotator cuff interval with arthroscopic correlation. Skeletal Radiol 2005;34:522–7.
18. Homsi C, Bordalo-Rodrigues M, da Silva J, et al. Ultrasound in adhesive capsulitis of the shoulder:

is assessment of the coracohumeral ligament a valuable diagnostic tool? Skeletal Radiol 2006; 35:673–8.

19. Strobel K, Zanetti M, Nagy L, et al. Suspected rotator cuff lesions: tissue harmonic imaging versus conventional US of the shoulder. Radiology 2004; 230:243–9.

20. Alasaarela E, Tervonen O, Takalo R, et al. Ultrasound evaluation of the acromioclavicular joint. J Rheumatol 1997;24:1954–63.

21. Blankstein A, Ganel A, Givon U, et al. Ultrasonography as a diagnostic modality in acromioclavicular joint pathologies. Isr Med Assoc J 2005;7: 28–30.

22. Hammond I. Unsuspected humeral head fracture diagnosed by ultrasound. J Ultrasound Med 1991; 10:422.

23. Prickett WD, Teefey SA, Galatz LM, et al. Accuracy of ultrasound imaging of the rotator cuff in shoulders that are painful postoperatively. J Bone Joint Surg Am 2003;85-A(6):1084–9.

24. Cole BJ, ElAttrache NS, Anbari A. Arthroscopic rotator cuff repairs: an anatomic and biomechanical rationale for different suture-anchor repair configurations. Arthroscopy 2007;23:662–9.

25. Crass JR, Craig EV, Feinberg SB. Sonography of the postoperative rotator cuff. AJR Am J Roentgenol 1986;146:561–4.

26. Mack LA, Nyberg DA, Matsen FA. Sonographic evaluation of the rotator cuff. Radiol Clin North Am 1988; 26:161–77.

27. Johal P, Martin D, Broadhurst N. Managing shoulder pain in general practice. Assessment, imaging and referral. Aust Fam Physician 2011;37:263–5.

Ultrasound of the Wrist and Hand

Ian Yu Yan TSOU, MBBS, FRCR (UK), MMed Imaging (Sydney)[a],*,
Jenn Nee KHOO, MB, BCh, BAO, FRCR (UK)[b]

KEYWORDS

• Ultrasound • Wrist • Hand • Finger • Thumb

KEY POINTS

- Because of the small anatomic size of the structures in the hand and wrist, the choice of high-frequency linear transducers with a small footprint is crucial.
- Excellent coupling can be achieved with the use of a water-bath, immersing the area of the fingers in water, without the need for ultrasound gel.
- Identification of the tendons and distinguishing them from one another is best done at the level of the wrist; then tracing and following the tendons distally.
- Tendons can show anisotropy, particularly in the volar flexor tendons within the finger. Appropriate angulation of the ultrasound probe is needed so as not to mistake this for a tear.
- The use of dynamic movement in flexion and extension of the fingers can provide useful information to the integrity of the tendon.

TECHNIQUE

The patient and sonographer should be seated opposite or 90° to each other, with the patient's hands resting on the examination table and supported by a pillow or rolled towel to expose the area of interest. High-frequency linear-array transducers (6–15 MHz) are essential; transducers with higher frequencies yield higher resolution, whereas those with lower frequencies afford better depth of penetration. A specialized transducer with a smaller footplate (2–3 cm), known as a hockey-stick because of the angle formed by the footplate and transducer handle, is frequently needed for its maneuverability around small joints. A coupling gel is required; the use of water bath for immersion of the fingers is becoming more widespread because there is no loss of sound-wave transmission even when there is loss of contact with the transducer in patients with fixed deformities and during dynamic assessment of finger tendon movement. The operator should be aware that these techniques are different or modified from those used when scanning other joints in the body.

In the hand and wrist, focused examinations targeted to answer the clinical question are usually performed. This includes scanning the relevant structures in at least two orthogonal planes, with dynamic and Doppler assessment. When in doubt, comparison can be made with the contralateral side.

ANATOMY
Sonographic Appearance

Tendons and ligaments are composed predominantly of sheets or bundles of Type I collagen fibers,[1] and appear as echogenic lines on longitudinal scans and dots on transverse scans. Tendon sheaths are seen as a thin echogenic layer surrounding the tendon, usually made more prominent when anechoic fluid is present within.

[a] Department of Diagnostic Radiology, Mount Elizabeth Hospital, 3 Mount Elizabeth, Singapore 228510, Republic of Singapore; [b] Department of Radiology, Changi General Hospital, 2 Simei Street 3, Singapore 529889, Republic of Singapore
* Corresponding author.
E-mail address: mrimaging@gmail.com

Ultrasound Clin 7 (2012) 439–455
http://dx.doi.org/10.1016/j.cult.2012.08.001
1556-858X/12/$ – see front matter © 2012 Elsevier Inc. All rights reserved

Although a small amount of tendon sheath fluid may be normal, tendon sheath thickening and vascularity is not. Fluid around ligaments, on the other hand, should alert the sonographer to careful interrogation for underlying pathologies.

Due to multiple parallel surfaces resulting from the sheet-like arrangement of their fibers, tendons and ligaments are frequently subject to anisotropy, which occurs when the transducer is not perpendicular to the scanned structure, causing the ultrasound (US) beam to be reflected away from the transducer. Loss of reflecting beam toward the transducer results in an erroneously hypoechoic appearance. This can be corrected simply by adjusting the transducer or rocking it along its longitudinal axis (heel-toeing).

Nerves are composed of bundles of fascicles contained within an epineurium. Each fascicle, in turn, is composed of multiple axons contained within a perineurium. On transverse scanning, this is seen as a collection of hypoechoic dots surrounded by the echogenic perineurium—all of which is encased in an echogenic epineurium.[2] This has been described as appearing like "a bunch of grapes."

Vessels can be easily identified by color Doppler signals. Whereas osseous structures are heavy reflectors of US waves, the cartilage-bone interface can be visualized as a smooth echogenic surface.

Wrist

Dorsal surface
The extensor compartments are formed by attachments from the overlying extensor retinaculum (a fibrous band stretching from the triquetrum and pisiform on the ulnar side to the anterior border of the distal radius) to the radius and ulna. Within each compartment is a single echogenic synovial sheath, containing their respective tendons (**Fig. 1**, **Table 1**).

The dorsal component of the scapholunate (SL) and lunotriquetral ligaments appear as fibrillar echogenic structures, whereas the triangular fibrocartilage (TFC) appears homogenously echogenic. The TFC is best assessed by placing the transducer along the ulnar side of the wrist in a paracoronal plane, using the extensor carpi ulnaris (ECU) tendon as the acoustic window. Although MR imaging remains the modality of choice to assess these structures, patients may present for US of a lump in these regions, which are revealed sonographically as ganglion cysts decompressing from tears of these structures.

Volar surface
The flexor tendons (**Fig. 2**) enter the wrist through the carpal tunnel, deep to the hypoechoic flexor retinaculum, which is attached to the pisiform and hook of hamate on the ulnar side and the scaphoid and trapezium on the radial side, where it splits into two laminae. The superficial band attaches to the scaphoid and trapezium tubercle, whereas the deep band attaches to the groove of the trapezium. The tendon of the flexor carpi radialis (FCR) traverses between these two bands. The flexor pollicis longus (FPL) is the most radially sited tendon within the carpal tunnel. The rest of the flexor tendons are contained within a single common compartment, with the flexor digitorum profundus (FDP) tendons deep to the flexor digitorum superficialis (FDS) tendons.

The median nerve lies just beneath the retinaculum, between the FPL on its radial side, and the FDS tendons on its ulnar side. As it traverses through the carpal tunnel, the nerve becomes progressively flatter. The normal cross-sectional area of the median nerve has been established at 10 mm^2 at the level of proximal margin of the retinaculum,[3] which is usually in the shape of an ellipse.

The ulnar nerve lies within Guyon canal, with the ulnar artery lateral to it. The pisiform and hamate forms the floor and the flexor retinaculum and pisohamate ligament forms the roof of Guyon canal.

The ulnar artery lies just superficial to the flexor retinaculum and the ulnar artery runs adjacent to the ulnar nerve.

Fingers

Extensor apparatus
The extensor tendons consist of extensor digitorum (ED), extensor indicis (EI), and extensor digiti minimi (EDM). There is significant anatomic variability in the arrangement of the extensor tendons. Most commonly, the ED provides one tendon slip to the index and middle finger, and two to the ring finger. The little finger receives two tendon slips from the EDM, which occasionally provides a tendon slip to the ring finger. The EI forms a single tendon that inserts into the extensor expansion at the metacarpal joint (MCPJ) of the index finger.

At the level of the MCPJ, the extensor tendons split into three slips which blend in with the extensor hood, a triangular fibrous expansion that appears as a thin (2 mm) echogenic structure. The central slip inserts into the dorsal aspect of the middle phalanx and is held in place by the sagittal band, a fibrous sheet that surrounds the MCPJ by inserting on either side of the volar plate. The two lateral slips receive contributions from the intrinsic muscles of the hands, converges into a conjoint

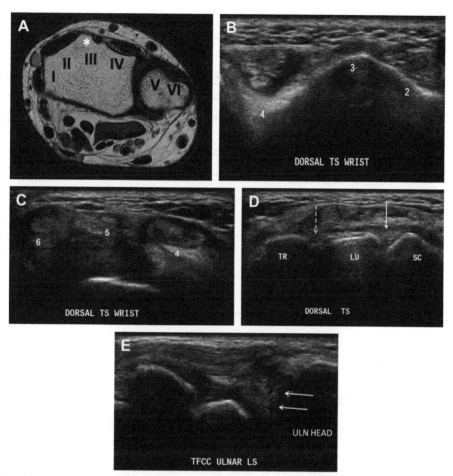

Fig. 1. (*A*) Axial T1-weighted MR imaging scan of the wrist extensor compartments I to VI. Acronyms are as listed in **Table 1**; Lister's tubercle (*asterisk*). (*B*) Corresponding US image of transverse section (TS) of second (2), third (3), and fourth (4) dorsal extensor compartments with the respective tendons in **Table 1**. (*C*) Corresponding US image of transverse section of fourth (4), fifth (5), and sixth (6) dorsal extensor compartments with the respective tendons in **Table 1**. (*D*) Transverse US image of the dorsal aspect of the wrist with the normal dorsal components of the scapholunate (*solid arrow*) and lunotriquetral (*dashed arrow*) ligaments, which connect the scaphoid (SC), lunate (LU) and triquetral (TR) bones. (*E*) Longitudinal section (LS) US image over the ulnar head (ULN HEAD) at the wrist with part of the articular disc of the triangular fibrocartilage complex (TFCC) (*arrows*), adjacent to the ulnar styloid process.

tendon at the level of the middle phalanx, and then inserts into the base of the distal phalanx.

Flexor surface

The flexor digitorum tendons continue along their respective digits in a similar arrangement as that in the wrist, until the proximal third of the proximal phalanx, where the FDS tendon splits into two slips, each passing around and reuniting deep to the FDP tendon, before attaching to the proximal half of the middle phalanx. The FDP tendon inserts at the base of the distal phalanx. The flexor tendons are divided into five zones (**Table 2**) based on anatomic considerations that have prognostic implications following tendon repair.[4]

The flexor tendons are held in place by its annular and cruciate pulley systems (**Table 3**). The annular pulleys consist of specific sites of focal thickening of the flexor synovial sheath and the cruciate pulleys are formed by additional crisscrossing fibers between the annular pulleys. The A2 pulley can be consistently seen with US, whereas the A4 pulley can be seen in slightly more than half the population. The rest of the pulleys cannot be visualized sonographically.[5] Sonographic depiction of the pulleys matches that of MR imaging[5,6] and has the added advantage of dynamic assessment.

The volar plate, a hypoechoic fibrocartilaginous structure, overlies the MCPJ and interphalangeal joints (IPJ). Distally, it has a broad-based attachment proximally and it divides into two slips known

Table 1
Summary of the anatomy of the extensor compartments of the wrist and its contents

Extensor Compartment	Tendons	Anatomic Landmark	Additional Notes
I	Abductor pollicis longus (APL) Extensor pollicis brevis (EPB)	Lateral to the radial styloid process	Occasionally contains a fibrous band separating the two tendons
II	Extensor carpi radialis longus (ECRL) Extensor carpi radialis brevis (ECRB)	Radial side of Lister's tubercle	—
III	Extensor pollicis longus (EPL)	Ulnar side of Lister's tubercle	Crosses tendons of compartment II
IV	Extensor digitorum (ED) Extensor indicis (EI)	—	—
V	Extensor digiti minimi (EDM)	—	—
VI	Extensor carpi ulnaris (ECU)	Between the head and styloid process of ulna	—

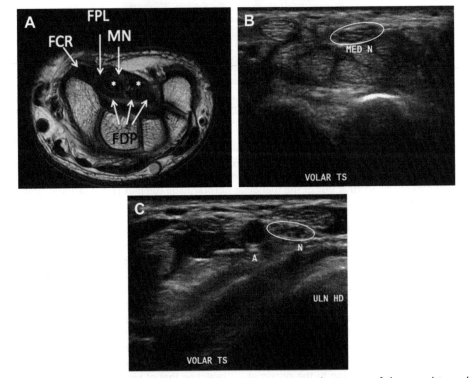

Fig. 2. (A) Axial T1-weighted MR imaging scan of the wrist contents and anatomy of the carpal tunnel. Flexor digitorum superficialis (asterisk). Abbreviations: FCR, flexor carpi radialis; FDP, flexor digitorum profundus; FPL, flexor pollicis longus; MN, median nerve. (B) Transverse US image of the carpal tunnel at the volar aspect of the wrist with the median nerve (MED N) (white oval) in the carpal tunnel with adjacent flexor tendons. The hypoechoic fascicles of the nerve can be distinguished. (C) Transverse US section at the level of the ulnar head (ULN HD); ulnar nerve (N) (white oval) adjacent to the ulnar artery (A).

Table 2
Summary of the anatomy of the flexor tendon zones

Flexor Tendon Zones	Second to Fourth Digits	First Digit
I	From finger tip to distal to insertion of FDS at middle phalanx (only contains FDP)	From finger tip to insertion of FPL (only contains FPL)
II	From A1 pulley to middle phalanx (the tendons pass through a restricted soft tissue space)	From neck of proximal phalanx to neck of metacarpal
III	From distal edge of carpal tunnel to A1 pulley	Thenar muscles
IV	Carpal tunnel	Carpal tunnel
V	From origins of tendons in the forearm to proximal border of carpal tunnel	From origins of tendons in the forearm to proximal border of carpal tunnel

as the check-rein ligaments that insert onto the neck of the metacarpal or phalanx.

Ligaments

Each MCPJ and IPJ is reinforced by the collateral ligaments, which course obliquely from posterolateral to anterolateral, inserting into the volar plate. They appear hypoechoic, fibrillar and convex.

Thumb

The anatomy of the thumb differs slightly from the other digits. On the ulnar side of the MCPJ, lies the adductor aponeurosis, an echogenic structure composed of fibers from the abductor pollicis longus (APL) and the extensor hood of the thumb. This inserts into the ulnar side of the base of the proximal phalanx, and lies superficial to the ulnar collateral ligament (UCL). Whether this relationship is preserved needs to be established when a UCL tear is present and this is usually examined from the dorsal surface. The insertion of the APL at

the dorsal aspect of the base of the first metacarpal can also be examined.

At the radial side of the first MCPJ, further tendinous insertions include that of opponens pollicis into the mid-to-distal first metacarpal, as well as abductor and flexor pollicis brevis into the base of the proximal phalanx. These are usually examined from the volar side.

PATHOLOGY
Traumatic Lesions

Tendon injuries

Tendon tears manifest as focal discontinuities,[7] with fluid or debris filling the gap between the tendon stumps (**Fig. 3**). When the gap is filled with debris, it may be difficult to distinguish partial tears from focal tendinopathies. However, in partial thickness tears, the tendon is usually attenuated (**Fig. 4**), whereas in tendinopathies the tendon is usually enlarged.[7] Increased tendon vascularity also favors tendinopathies.

Table 3
Summary of the annular and cruciate pulley systems

Pulleys	Location (Fingers)	Location (Thumb)
A1	Volar plate of MCPJ to base of proximal phalanx	MCPJ
A2	Proximal part of proximal phalanx to junction between the middle and distal third of proximal phalanx	DIPJ
A3	Proximal interphalangeal joint	—
A4	Midshaft of middle phalanx	—
A5	Distal interphalangeal joint	—
C1	Between A2 and A3	—
C2	Between A3 and A4	—
C3	Between A4 and A5	—

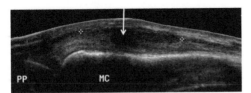

Fig. 3. Panoramic longitudinal section of a tendon gap (*white arrow*) with a few remnant fibers, in keeping with a partial tear. Cross markers delineate the areas of tendinopathy, overlying the metacarpal (MC), proximal phalanx (PP).

When a flexor tendon tear is suspected, a thorough clinical examination of its functional deficit frequently helps direct the US examination. An FDP tear will manifest as inability to actively flex the distal IPJ, with preserved flexion of the proximal IPJ (PIPJ). Tendon excursion during dynamic assessment reflects functionality. The direction of tendon excursion should also be congruent with the direction of passive movement, which can be controlled by the sonographer. The extent of tendon retraction should be evaluated because this has important implications if surgical repair is being considered.

The most frequently torn extensor tendon is the extensor pollicis longus (EPL). This may be related

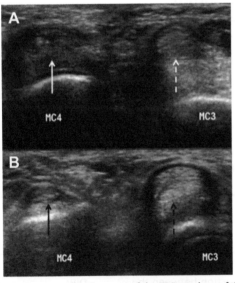

Fig. 4. Transverse section scan of the FDP tendons of the ring finger (MC4) and middle finger (MC3) at the level of the MCPJ (*A*) and distal to the MCPJ (*B*). (*A*) Disorganized and heterogeneous appearance of the FDP tendon of MC4 (*solid white arrow*) is in keeping with a chronic partial tear with scarring. Normal appearance of FDP and FDS of MC3 (*broken white arrow*). (*B*) The flexor tendon complex of MC4 is attenuated due to the tear (*solid black arrow*) compared with the normal girth of the flexor tendon complex of MC3 (*broken black arrow*).

to rheumatologic conditions, wrist trauma, or be spontaneous. It is thought that the tendon may be more prone to tears at the Lister's tubercle because of the vascular watershed nature of this region. In suspected EPL tears arising from compression from fixation plates of wrist fractures, US is the modality of choice because of the limitations of MR imaging from susceptibility resulting from the orthopedic hardware (Fig. 5). The EI should always be evaluated as a potential graft donor.

Flexor tendon injuries are less common. The location of the injury is an important prognostic factor. Zone 2 and 5 injuries have significantly poorer outcome postoperatively because there is a propensity for adhesions due to the restricted soft tissue space through which the tendons traverse.[8]

US is able to demonstrate postoperative complications, such as suture dehiscence with retear (Fig. 6) and entrapment by scar tissue. Repaired tendons usually appear heterogeneous with ill-defined margins, whereas suture materials will appear echogenic with faint reverberation artifacts.

Ligament injuries

Although collateral ligaments injuries can be demonstrated on MR imaging, the substantially shorter examination time of US scans is a significant advantage. Tiny avulsion fragments, which may be difficult to detect on radiographs and MR imaging, are seen as brightly echogenic foci (Fig. 7). In UCL tears of the first MCPJ, the location of the torn ligament stump relative to the adductor aponeurosis needs to be carefully evaluated (Fig. 8). When the torn ligament is flipped superficial to the adductor aponeurosis (Stener lesion), surgical repair is indicated.

Tendon instability

Tendon instabilities result from injury to the reinforcing structures, namely the flexor pulley systems, extensor hoods, and wrist retinacula. Dynamic US assessment demonstrates these injuries elegantly.

Injuries to the flexor tendon pulley system, whose primary function is to convert linear translation forces into rotational forces and torque at the joints, may also present with limitation of finger flexion. The A2 and A4 pulleys seem to be the most important. Injuries of the pulleys occur in a predictable manner, with disruption usually occurring at the A2 pulley, progressing to the A3, A4, and occasionally, A1 pulley.[9] A recent study by Hauger and colleagues[5] found that US and MR imaging detection of direct signs of A2 and A4 pulley injuries is equally matched. The pulleys serve to hold the tendon close to or against the phalanges on flexion of the finger. Bow-stringing of the flexor tendons, in which the tendon pulls

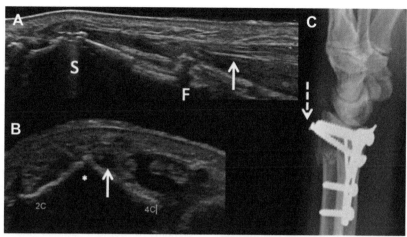

Fig. 5. (A) Panoramic longitudinal scan of the dorsal surface of the wrist with discontinuity of EPL, with its retracted stump (*white arrow*) at the level of the fracture site (F). Protrusion of the screw (S) beyond the cortical margin of the distal radius. (B) Corresponding TS scan with absence of the EPL tendon (*white arrow*) at its usual location adjacent to Lister's tubercle (*asterisk*). *Abbreviations:* 2C, second extensor compartment; 4C, fourth extensor compartment. (C) Lateral radiograph of the wrist with protrusion of the metallic screw into the soft tissues of the dorsal aspect of the wrist (*broken arrow*).

away from the underlying bone on flexion of the finger, is a classical secondary sign of pulley ruptures, and can be seen on both US and MR imaging, although US offers the added advantage of dynamic assessment, in which bow-stringing is exaggerated by forced finger flexion against resistance.

Sagittal band rupture (**Fig. 9**), also known as boxer's knuckle, is inferred by dislocation of the

extensor tendon, which, again, is exaggerated with finger flexion. It is more commonly torn on its radial side, resulting in ulnar subluxation of the tendon.[10] Pathologic studies have shown that the radial sagittal band is often longer and thinner than its ulnar counterpart is, possibly explaining its propensity to tears.[11]

In the wrist, the most common tendon instability is that of ECU, due to disruption of the retinaculum from its ulnar attachment. Repetitive stress from sudden pronation in tennis players and pannus disruption in rheumatoid arthritis are two of the most common causes. In ECU instability, the tendon will dislocate into the volar surface of the ulna.

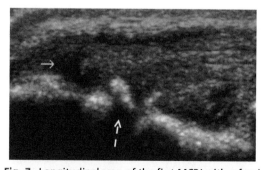

Fig. 6. Longitudinal scans at the level of the MCPJ (A) and proximal phalanx (B) of a patient with surgical repair of ED. Echogenic material representing sutures are labeled as 'proximal sutures' at the level of the MCPJ and 'distal sutures' at the level of the proximal phalanx. (A) The retracted tendon stump is seen proximal to proximal sutures (*broken white arrows*), while distal to it, irregular soft tissue material is seen (*block arrows*). (B) Nonvisualization of tendon material with irregular soft tissue filling the tendon gap between the proximal and distal sutures (*block arrows*).

Fig. 7. Longitudinal scan of the first MCPJ with a focal anechoic gap at the phalangeal insertion of the UCL (*solid white arrow*), in keeping with a complete tear. This is associated with focal cortical break at the adjacent base of the proximal phalanx (*broken white arrow*), in keeping with a tiny avulsed fracture fragment.

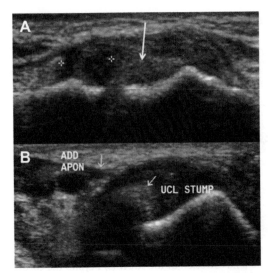

Fig. 8. Longitudinal section (A) and transverse section (B) scans of the ulnar aspect of the 1st MCPJ. (A) The UCL is discontinuous at its phalangeal insertion (cross markers), in keeping with a tear. Echogenic retracted UCL stump (white arrow). (B) Normal relationship of the UCL stump and adductor aponeurosis (ADD APON) is preserved. The echogenic torn UCL stump remains deep to the hypoechoic adductor aponeurosis (arrows).

Foreign body

Sonography is also extremely useful for detection of radiolucent foreign bodies (Fig. 10), which appear strongly echogenic, occasionally with reverberation artifacts. Often, the foreign bodies involving the hand and wrist are of relatively small size and may not be seen on MR imaging. Chronically embedded foreign bodies may also lead to formation of epidermal inclusion cysts, and sonographic demonstration of the foreign body within the mass is virtually pathognomonic.

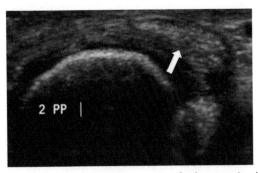

Fig. 9. Transverse section scan of the proximal phalanx of the index finger (2 PP). Tear of the radial sagittal band is inferred from ulnar dislocation of the echogenic extensor tendon (white arrow).

DEGENERATIVE OR OVERUSE PATHOLOGIES

The wrists and hands are frequently subject to overuse and degenerative conditions. Repetitive friction leads to inflammation and, eventually, fibrosing degeneration or degenerative tears. Degenerative tendon and ligament tears are similar in appearance to traumatic tears.

De Quervain Tenosynovitis

When the tendon sheath of the first extensor compartment is affected, it is known as De Quervain tenosynovitis. This is usually seen as fluid within a thickened tendon sheath and is frequently associated with underlying tendinopathy. Occasionally, a septum divides the first extensor compartment into two subtunnels, with only the EPB demonstrating tendinosis. This is a clinically significant variant that affects treatment planning and outcome, be it surgical[12] or US-guided injections of antiinflammatory agents.[13]

Trigger Finger or Thumb

Trigger finger or thumb is a common affliction, particularly in middle-aged women, and clinically presents with transient locking of a flexed digit and painful snapping during extension. This most commonly affects the A1 pulley. US findings include thickening of the pulley (Fig. 11), wasting of the tendon with tendinosis, and loss of the normal smooth gliding movement of the tendon. On active movement, correlation with catching of the tendon on US to a palpable click is highly suggestive of trigger finger.

Intersection Syndromes

The proximal intersection syndrome refers to friction between the myotendinous junctions of the first extensor compartment tendons with the second, and is a common differential diagnosis for de Quervain disease. The lesser-known distal intersection syndrome involves the crossover of the second and third extensor compartment tendons beyond Lister's tubercle (Fig. 12).

Intrinsic Ligaments of the Wrist and Triangular Fibrocartilage

Several studies evaluating sonographic ability to detect tears of the dorsal SL ligament and TFC have shown promising results. Keogh and colleagues[14] showed that sonographic findings of TFC tears correlated with MR imaging and arthroscopy in more than 80% of cases, with the tears appearing as hypoechoic disruptions of the normally echogenic TFC.

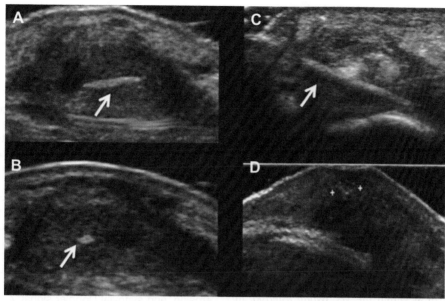

Fig. 10. US scans with a variety of radiolucent foreign bodies, confirmed surgically. (*A, B*) Longitudinal and transverse section scan appearance of a wooden splinter (*white arrow*) surrounded by hypoechoic granulation tissue. (*C*) Longitudinal section of a wooden splinter adjacent to a tendon (*white arrow*). (*D*) Longitudinal section scan of glass shards (*cross markers*).

Taljanovic and colleagues[15] demonstrated 94% accuracy in sonographic detection of dorsal band SL ligament tears compared with MR arthrogram. US performed less well with regard to lunotriquetral ligament tears, with only 75% accuracy. Again, these are demonstrated on US as disruptions of their normally echogenic fibers.

These early results are certainly encouraging because targeted US of these regions is quick and cheap to perform. In many centers, however, MR imaging is still the norm for evaluation of patients with wrist pain. Regardless, one should still be familiar with the normal and pathologic appearance of these structures because wrist lumps in patients presenting for US scans may represent ganglion cysts decompressing from these tears (**Figs. 13** and **14**).

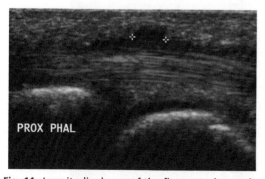

Fig. 11. Longitudinal scan of the flexor tendon at the level of the MCPJ with thickening of the A1 pulley (*cross markers*), resulting in trigger finger.

Osseous Degeneration

Articular degenerative changes are demonstrated as irregularities of the cartilage-bone interface with marginal osteophytes (**Fig. 15**). Impingement of the adjacent tendons by osteophytes may result in tenosynovitis, tendinopathies, and tears. This is

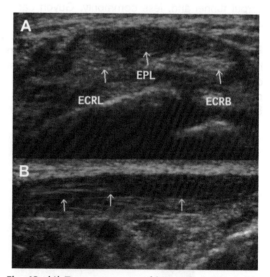

Fig. 12. (*A*) Transverse scan of hypoechoic EPL (*white arrows*) with a small amount of tendon sheath fluid, in keeping with tendinosis and tenosynovitis, as it crosses extensor carpi radialis longus (ECRL) and extensor carpi radialis brevis (ECRB). (*B*) Longitudinal scan of a hypoechoic EPL (*white arrows*) as it crosses over the second extensor compartment.

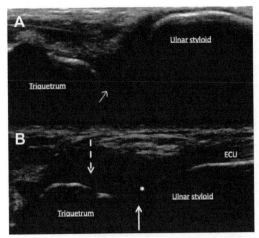

Fig. 13. (A) Longitudinal scan in coronal orientation of the normal echogenic TFC (*white arrow*) between the ulnar styloid and triquetrum. (B) Longitudinal scan in coronal orientation of a hypoechoic gap (*solid white arrow*) at within the TFC (*white asterisk*), in keeping with a tear. A small ganglion cyst (*broken white arrow*) is seen decompressing from the TFC tear.

most commonly seen in triscaphe osteoarthritis with resultant FCR pathologies. The main role of US is to exclude a ganglion cyst because these patients frequently present with a painful lump.

ENTRAPMENT NEUROPATHIES

Entrapment neuropathies in the wrists consist of carpal tunnel and, less commonly, Guyon canal syndromes.

Carpal tunnel syndrome refers to entrapment and swelling of the median nerve, resulting in an enlarged hypoechoic median nerve on US (**Fig. 16**). Most carpal tunnel syndromes are idiopathic. However, occasionally, other causes, such as pannus formation from rheumatoid arthritis or mass effect from

space-occupying lesions, may be demonstrated on US. Guyon canal syndrome may be caused by chronic repetitive external pressure, space-occupying lesions, or be secondary to fractures.

INFLAMMATORY ARTHRITIDES

US is playing an increasingly important role in the diagnosis and management of patients with inflammatory arthritides. It is far superior to radiography in detection of early disease, and disease progression and therapeutic response can be monitored with serial US. Although there is evidence that MR imaging may be superior in disease detection and monitoring, US is preferred in many centers because it is less time-consuming and cost-intensive.

Four sonographic criteria with individual grading systems have been established by OMERACT[16]: joint effusion, synovial hypertrophy, osseous erosion, and synovial Doppler signal. A joint effusion is characterized by intraarticular hypoechoic or anechoic signal, which is displaceable and compressible. Synovial hypertrophy is defined as hypoechoic, intraarticular, nondisplaceable, and poorly compressible soft tissue.

Osseous erosion is characterized by intraarticular discontinuity of a bony surface that is visible in two orthogonal planes (**Fig. 17**). Through sound transmission with adjacent active synovitis indicates an acute erosion. Normal anatomic cortical depressions in the dorsal aspect of the metacarpal head should not be mistaken for erosions.

Synovial Doppler signal is defined as color spots corresponding to areas of increased synovial perfusion and/or angiogenesis. This differentiates active synovitis from inactive pannus and debris (**Fig. 18**). Both Power Doppler US (PDUS) and color flow Doppler US (CFDUS) can be used. PDUS has a broader dynamic range and better

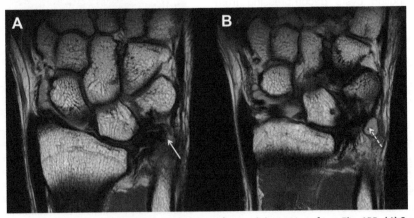

Fig. 14. Corresponding sequential coronal proton density images of the patient from **Fig. 13**B. (A) Small gap in the TFC (*solid white arrow*) in keeping with a tear. (B) Small ganglion cyst (*broken arrow*) decompressing from the tear.

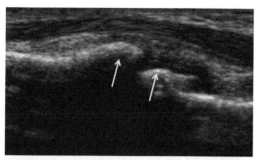

Fig. 15. Longitudinal scan at the level of the PIPJ of protruding cortical outgrowths (*arrows*), in keeping with osteophytes from osteoarthritis.

flow sensitivity. It is also angle independent and unaffected by aliasing. Low pulse repetition frequency and small region of interest maximizes the detection of vascularity within the synovium, whereas reducing the gain settings reduces interface artifact. PDUS findings have been found to correlate well with pathologic changes of active synovitis. PDUS quantification is based on the amount of color pixels visualized, whereas CFDUS yields a pressure trace from which the resistive index may be calculated, allowing for a more objective measure of synovitis. Despite this, PDUS is still preferred over CFDUS because of its higher sensitivity.

Rheumatoid Arthritis

A chronic inflammatory systemic disease of unknown cause, rheumatoid arthritis most commonly affects the joints, with chronic synovitis and pannus formation leading to chondral and osseous destruction. Significant morbidity and mortality has been associated with it and the current cornerstone of management is early detection, with early commencement and modification of therapy. Radiographic demonstration of erosions is now considered advanced disease and emphasis is now on early detection of synovitis.

Sonography plays a pivotal role in both disease detection and monitoring and has become an extension of the clinical examination for many rheumatologists.

PDUS signal is a sensitive and accurate indication of active disease,[17] whereas pannus is seen as a periarticular heterogeneous mass continuous with the hypertrophied synovium (**Fig. 19**). Erosions are most frequently seen in the radial aspects of the metacarpals heads and phalangeal bases, usually those of the second, third, and fifth digits.[18] US is able to detect erosions 1 to 2 years before their radiographic appearance.[19]

Depositional Arthropathy

A variety of crystals can aggregate in joints, leading to acute or chronic arthritis. Gouty arthropathy is the most common, in which monosodium urate crystals are deposited on the surface of hyaline cartilages. These are seen as irregular hyperechoic bands overlying the hypoechoic cartilage, described as the double-contour sign. Recent studies[20] have shown that this can be demonstrated in 92% of patients with gout. Tophaceous gout is also easily seen on US (**Fig. 20**). Other depositional arthropathies include calcium pyrophosphate dihydrate deposition disease (pseudogout), in which the crystals are deposited within the cartilage.[20] Distinguishing between the different types of depositional arthropathies may not be essential in the acute setting because the initial treatment does not differ significantly. However, urate-lowering drugs remain the mainstay of long-term therapy for patients with gout and US may obviate the need of needle aspiration for joint fluid analysis, which carries a small but significant risk of infection.

INFECTIVE ARTHRITIS

Although US is able to demonstrate inflammatory synovitis and effusion, septic arthritis remains

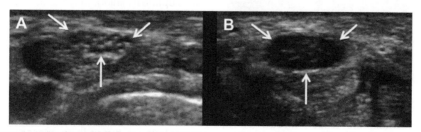

Fig. 16. Transverse scans through the carpal tunnel of two patients. (*A*) Normal bunch-of-grapes appearance of the median nerve (*arrows*). (*B*) Hypoechoic enlarged median nerve (*arrows*) in keeping with carpal tunnel syndrome.

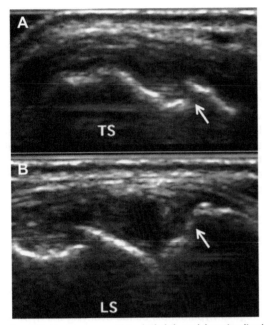

Fig. 17. Transverse section (TS) (*A*) and longitudinal section (LS) (*B*) scans of cortical discontinuity in the metacarpal head in orthogonal planes, in keeping with osseous erosion (*white arrows*).

a clinical diagnosis because it cannot be differentiated from other forms of early inflammatory arthritides. In patients whose effusions are small and clinically difficult to elicit, US may also be used to assist diagnostic joint aspirations.

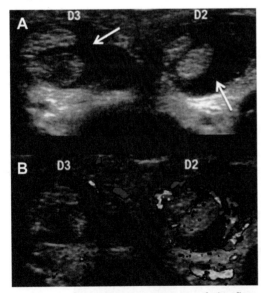

Fig. 18. (*A*) Grayscale transverse scan of the flexor tendons of the 2nd (D2) and 3rd (D3) digits with anechoic fluid within the tendon sheaths (*arrow*, D3), with areas of hypoechoic thickening (*arrow*, D2). (*B*) Doppler TS scan of marked tendon sheath vascularity of D2 indicating active tenosynovitis.

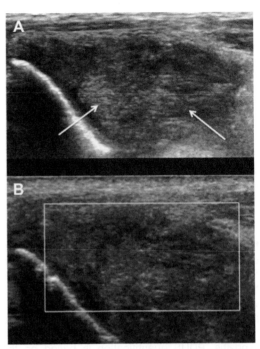

Fig. 19. (*A*) Grayscale longitudinal scan of the wrist of a rheumatoid patient with a large periarticular mass (*white arrow*). (*B*) Doppler longitudinal scan with absence of vascularity (*box*) indicating inactive disease.

SPACE-OCCUPYING LESIONS

Although US can reliably differentiate cystic from solid masses, very few lesions have specific US appearances and, frequently, further MR imaging or histologic evaluation is eventually required. However, useful information about anatomic relationships and vascularity of the lesion may be gleaned sonographically. This is useful for surgical planning.

The most common mass in the wrists and hands is a ganglion, usually arising from joints and tendon sheaths. Its exact cause remains unknown, but it is widely believed to represent degeneration of mucoid connective tissue. Although histologically it differs from a synovial cyst in that it possesses a myxoid wall with no true epithelial lining, they cannot be differentiated sonographically, with both appearing as well-defined anechoic or hypoechoic cystic masses, depending on the contents. Occasionally, a neck arising from the adjacent joint can be identified. When tubular, it needs to be differentiated from vascular structures (**Fig. 21**).

Vascular malformations (**Figs. 22** and **23**) are generally demonstrated as compressible solid hyperechoic or hypoechoic masses, occasionally with serpiginous components. Dilated feeding and draining vessels may be demonstrated, as

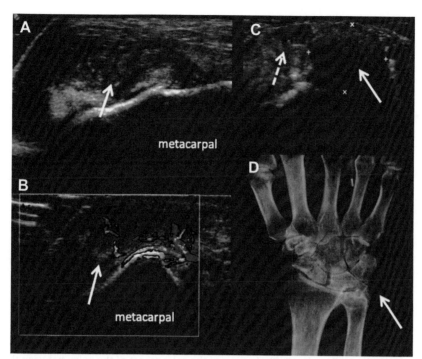

Fig. 20. (*A*) Longitudinal scan at the level of the MCPJ of a patient with gout with heterogeneous periarticular soft tissue, in keeping with a tophus (*white arrows*). (*B*) TS scan of the same patient with significant vascularity (*arrow*), indicating active inflammation. (*C*) TS scan at the level of the wrist of a different patient with the tophus (*solid arrow*) adjacent to the median nerve (*broken arrow*). Space-occupying lesions can potentially cause carpal tunnel syndrome. (*D*) Corresponding frontal wrist radiograph of the same patient with characteristic periarticular erosions typical of gout (*arrow*).

well as internal arterial flow. Absence of internal flow, however, does not exclude vascular malformations because cavernous types may contain slow flow, which may not be detectable on US.

Giant cell tumors of the tendon sheaths (known as pigmented villonodular synovitis when they occur elsewhere) are the second most common space-occupying lesions encountered in this

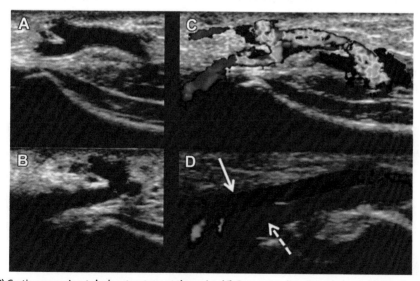

Fig. 21. (*A*, *B*) Cystic-appearing tubular structure at the wrist. (*C*) Corresponding Doppler scan bidirectional flow within it, in keeping with an arteriovenous fistula. (*D*) Longitudinal Doppler scan of a different patient with a tubular anechoic structure without color flow (*broken arrow*) adjacent to a vessel (*solid arrow*), confirming a cystic structure, likely to be a ganglion cyst.

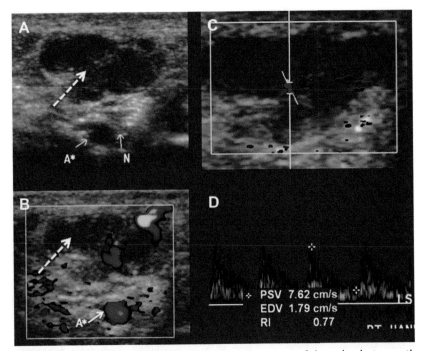

Fig. 22. Grayscale US (*A*) and Doppler (*B–D*) of a mass at the volar aspect of the palm, between the 2nd and 3rd metacarpals; vascular in nature. (*A*) TS scan of a lobulated hypoechoic mass (*broken white arrow*), with the neurovascular bundle (*A*, vessel; N, nerve*) just beneath it. (*B*) Doppler scan of color flow within the mass and the tubular structure just beneath it (*broken arrow*), in keeping with a vessel (*A**). (*C, D*) Internal arterial flow.

region. Although these are histologically benign, they can enlarge to cause significant osseous erosion and destruction. They are usually found on the volar surface of the finger, at or distal to the PIPJ, and appear as well-defined hypoechoic solid masses with internal vascularity.

The finger is the most common site for a glomus tumor even though, by itself, a glomus tumor is uncommon. It is a benign hamartoma arising from the neuromyoarterial glomus body, which is believed to play a role in thermoregulation and is found in higher concentrations in the fingertips. Although its sonographic appearance ranges from nonspecific soft tissue thickening to a circumscribed hypoechoic mass, avid vascularity and its typical location points to a glomus tumor (**Fig. 24**).

Space-occupying lesions arising from neural structures are also commonly seen (**Fig. 25**). Peripheral nerve sheath tumors are recognized by their fusiform shape and target sign. Schwannomas may occasionally be differentiated from neurofibromas by their eccentric location. Rare neural

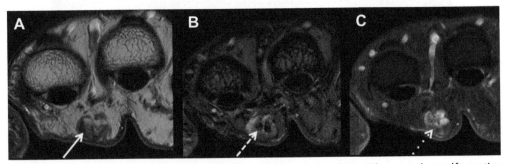

Fig. 23. MR imaging scan of the same mass in **Fig. 22** of features in keeping with a vascular malformation. (*A*) Axial proton density scan of a lobulated heterogeneous mass (*solid white arrow*). (*B*) Axial gradient-recalled scan of foci of susceptibility within it (*broken white arrow*), indicating blood products. (*C*) Axial postcontrast fat-saturated T1-weighted scan of heterogeneous enhancement of the mass (*dotted white arrow*).

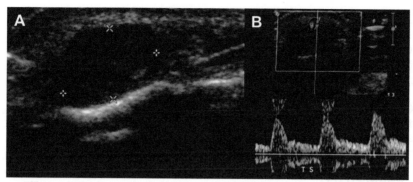

Fig. 24. (*A*) Transverse scan of a well-defined hypoechoic mass within the subcutaneous tissue (*cross markers*). (*B*) Corresponding Doppler scan of avid internal vascularity with arterial flow and aliasing artifact.

masses include fibrolipomatous hamartoma, which most commonly affect the medial nerve and demonstrate sonographically pathognomonic appearances of neural enlargement with echogenic fatty tissue interspersed between normal-appearing hypoechoic neural fascicles. Trauma to the nerves may result in scarring and also present as a mass.

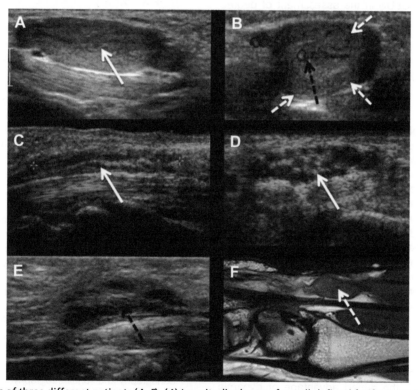

Fig. 25. Scans of three different patients (*A–F*). (*A*) Longitudinal scan of a well-defined fusiform mass in the palm (*white arrow*). (*B*) Transverse scan of 'target sign, with peripheral hypoechogenicity (*broken white arrows*) and central hyperechogenicity (*broken black arrow*, which is also pointing to Doppler signal), in keeping with a benign peripheral nerve sheath tumor. (*C*) Longitudinal scan of thickening of the median nerve (*white arrow*) at the level of the volar aspect of the wrist. (*D*) Transverse scan of characteristic echogenic fat between normal hypoechoic neural fascicles, in keeping with a fibrolipomatous hamartoma (*white arrow*). (*E*) Longitudinal scan of focal thickening and disruption of the median nerve (*broken arrow*), at the level volar to the distal radius, in keeping with scarring from prior trauma. (*F*) Sagittal proton density MR image of nonspecific thickening of the median nerve (*broken arrow*), with a similar configuration.

Malignant Masses

Malignant lesions of the hands and wrists are uncommon. Occasionally, soft tissue sarcomas or metastases may be found. US appearance of malignant masses is nonpathognomonic, and they are usually seen as hypoechoic masses with internal vascularity. Of note, a simple lipoma cannot be distinguished from a well-differentiated liposarcoma sonographically, with both appearing as well-defined lobulated hyperechoic masses.

CONTRAST-ENHANCED US

Contrast-enhanced US (CEUS) has garnered significant interest in the recent years. Patients who were previously contraindicated for intravenous CT or MR contrast now have a viable option. The lack of radiation of CEUS has also allowed for research in more creative uses of contrast imaging. Currently, the European Federation of Societies for Ultrasound in Medicine and Biology (EFSUMB) guidelines[21] suggest that there may be a role of CEUS in the assessment of degree of vascularity in rheumatoid arthritis, serving as a more sensitive marker of disease activity and therapeutic response.

ULTRASOUND-GUIDED INTERVENTIONS

The advent of new generation high-frequency transducers and improved US software have led to significant improvements in image resolution and this, in turn, has allowed for greater advances in musculoskeletal intervention. The advantage of real-time assessment and direct visualization allows for accurate needle placement and observation of therapeutic delivery, conferring a greater degree of confidence to the interventionist. Simple US-guided drainages and injections may be performed at the bedside or in the clinic. Tendon peritendinous injections of antiinflammatory agents and removal of small foreign bodies may also be performed under US guidance.

SUMMARY

The small joints of the hands and wrists are amenable to both MR imaging and US imaging. Apart from the lower cost and shorter examination time, US has the added advantage of dynamic assessment of the joints and is gaining favor among many clinicians and radiologists alike.

REFERENCES

1. Vigorita VJ. Soft tissue pathology. In: Orthopaedic pathology. 2nd edition. Philadelphia: Lippincott Williams & Wilkins; 2008. p. 711.
2. Silvestri E, Martinoli C, Derchi LE, et al. Echotexture of peripheral nerves: correlation between US and histologic findings and criteria to differentiate tendons. Radiology 1995;197:291–6.
3. Ziswiler HR, Reichen bach S, Vogelin E, et al. Diagnostic value of sonography in patients with suspected carpal tunnel syndrome: a prospective study. Arthritis Rheum 2005;52(1):304–11.
4. Verdan CE. Primary repair of flexor tendons. J Bone Joint Surg Am 1960;42-A:647–57.
5. Hauger O, Chung CB, Lektrakul N, et al. Pulley system in the fingers: normal anatomy and simulated lesions in cadavers at MR imaging, CT, and US with and without contrast material distention of the tendon sheath. Radiology 2000;217:201–12.
6. Martinoli C, Bianchi S, Nebiolo M, et al. Sonographic evaluation of digital annular pulley tears. Skeletal Radiol 2000;29:387–91.
7. Van Holsbeeck MT, Introcaso JH. Sonography of tendons. In: Musculoskeletal ultrasound. 2nd edition. Missouri: Mosby; 2000. p. 77–129.
8. Beasley RW. Tendon injuries. In: Gumpert E, editor. Beasley's surgery of the hand. New York: Thieme Medical Publishers, Inc; 2003. p. 239.
9. Marco RA, Sharkey NA, Smith TS, et al. Pathomechanics of closed rupture of the flexor tendon pulley in rock climbers. J Bone Joint Surg Am 1998;80(7):1012–9.
10. Watson HK, Weinzweig J, Guidera PM. Sagittal band reconstruction. J Hand Surg Am 1997;22(3):452–6.
11. Rayan GM, Murray D, Chung KW, et al. The extensor retinacular system at the metacarpophalangeal joint. Anatomical and histological study. J Hand Surg Br 1997;22(5):585–90.
12. Giles KW. Anatomical variations affecting the surgery of de Quervain's disease. J Bone Joint Surg Br 1960;42-B:352–5.
13. Witt J, Pess G, Gelberman RH. Treatment of de Quervain tenosynovitis. A prospective study of the results of injection of steroids and immobilization in a splint. J Bone Joint Surg Am 1991;73(2):219–22.
14. Keogh CF, Wong AD, Wells NJ, et al. High-resolution sonography of the triangular fibrocartilage: initial experience and correlation with MRI and arthroscopic findings. AJR Am J Roentgenol 2004;182(2):333–6.
15. Taljanovic MS, Sheppard JE, Jones MD, et al. Sonography and sonoarthrographyc of the scapholunate and lunotriquetrial ligaments and triangular fibrocartilage disk: initial experience and correlation with arthrography and magnetic resonance arthrography. J Ultrasound Med 2008;27(2):179–91.
16. Wakefield RJ, Balint PV, Szkudlarek M, et al. Musculoskeletal ultrasound including definitions for ultrasonographic pathology. J Rheumatol 2005;32(2):2485–7.

17. The J, Stevens K, Williamson L, et al. Power Doppler ultrasound of rheumatoid synovitis: quantification of therapeutic response. Br J Radiol 2003;76(912):875–9.

18. McNally EG. Ultrasound of the small joints of the hands and feet: current status. Skeletal Radiol 2008;37(2):99–113.

19. Backhaus M, Burmester GR, Sandrock D, et al. Prospective two year follow up study comparing novel and conventional imaging procedures in patients with arthritic finger joints. Ann Rheum Dis 2006;61:895–904.

20. Thiele RG, Schlesinger N. Diagnosis of gout by ultrasound. Rheumatology (Oxford) 2007;46(7):1116–21.

21. Albrecht T, Blomley M, Bolondi L, et al. Guidelines for the use of contrast agents in ultrasound. 2004. Available at: http://www.efsumb.org/guidelines/efsumb-guidelines-ceus.pdf. Accessed March 23. 2012.

Ultrasonography of the Hip and Groin: Sports Injuries and Hernias

Howard Pinchcofsky, MD[a],*,
Gervais Khin-Lin Wansaicheong, MBBS, FRCR, MMed (Diagnostic Radiology)[b]

KEYWORDS

- Musculoskeletal ultrasonography • Groin • Joint effusion • Tendinosis • Hernia • Mesh

KEY POINTS

- Ultrasonography of the hip and groin is more effective than other modalities when imaging metal.
- The anterior hip structures most commonly associated with sports injuries include the tensor fascia lata tendon and the rectus femoris near the aponeurosis.
- Injuries to the gluteus medius and minimus tendons are largely dependent on demographics.
- The adductor longus is the hip adductor most commonly injured in athletes.
- The patient should be examined for hernias in the supine and upright positions.
- Diagnosis of direct and indirect hernias depends on the relationship of the neck of the hernia sac to the inferior epigastric artery.

 Videos of groin anatomy during coughing and at rest, including small hernia, accompany this article.

SPORTS INJURIES
Introduction

Ultrasonography is an effective method of evaluating sports injuries of the groin. The quality of the ultrasound transducers available with modern ultrasound units has advanced to such an extent that fine anatomic detail can be easily assessed. The internal echotexture of muscles, tendons, and nerves is readily apparent. The ability to characterize joint effusions with ultrasonography from simple to complex is a major advantage of ultrasonography over other imaging modalities. Ultrasonography has superior spatial resolution compared with magnetic resonance (MR), such that tendons and nerves are easily followed, and the location of lesions such as neuromas or tendon tears can be accurately described. Dynamic evaluation of anatomic structures is available with ultrasonography, which often adds a significant amount of information to the imaging diagnosis. Many patients who have orthopedic hardware or metallic foreign material in the region of interest would benefit from sonographic evaluation because sound waves do not produce artifacts that interact with metal to distort or mask the surrounding anatomic structures. Ultrasonography can image nonradiopaque foreign material such as wood, which is an advantage over radiography and computed tomography (CT). Patients who are claustrophobic or have difficulty lying still can be imaged by ultrasonography with a much better result than with MR or CT.

Funding sources. None. Conflict of interest: None.
[a] Department of Diagnostic Radiology, Union Hospital of Cecil County, 106 Bow St, Elkton, MD 21921, USA;
[b] Department of Diagnostic Radiology, Tan Tock Seng Hospital, Singapore 308433
* Corresponding author.
E-mail address: hpinchcofsky@uhcc.com

Ultrasound Clin 7 (2012) 457–473
http://dx.doi.org/10.1016/j.cult.2012.08.002
1556-858X/12/$ – see front matter © 2012 Elsevier Inc. All rights reserved.

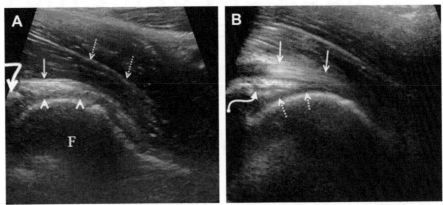

Fig. 1. Longitudinal evaluation of the hip demonstrating normal anatomy. (*A*) Acetabulum (*curved arrow*), femoral head (F), anterior-superior labrum (*solid arrow*), iliopsoas muscle (*dashed arrows*), and articular cartilage (*arrowheads*). (*B*) Anterior-superior labrum (*curved arrow*) with incidental tear, iliopsoas tendon (*solid arrows*), and hypoechoic hyaline cartilage (*dashed arrows*).

The optimal transducer frequency to evaluate the hip region varies depending on the size of the patient. Transducer frequency usually varies between 5 and 12 MHz, but can be as low as 3.5 MHz if there is a large amount of soft tissue to be penetrated.[1–3] Linear transducers are used most of the time; however, in very large patients, curvilinear probes are often necessary for adequate penetration. As with any ultrasound examination, adjusting the scanning depth and the location of the focal zone are paramount to achieving good results. Sonographic evaluation of the hip is divided into 4 parts: anterior (including the hip joint), lateral, medial, and posterior. A general principle of evaluation of all of these compartments is that all anatomic structures should be assessed in both the transverse plane and the long axis. Dynamic evaluations and imaging with color or power Doppler should always be used when deemed necessary by the operator. Communication with the patient is important while scanning, as the patient's symptoms will often focus the examination to the region of interest. The first part of this article describes the anterior, lateral, medial, and posterior parts of the hip and groin, and serves to acquaint the reader with normal and abnormal sonographic findings.

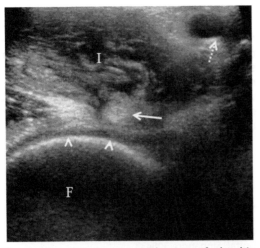

Fig. 2. Normal transverse evaluation of the hip. Femoral head (F), iliopsoas tendon (*solid arrow*), iliopsoas muscle (I), hyaline cartilage (*arrowheads*), and femoral vessels (*dashed arrow*).

Box 1
Anatomic structures that should be identified during longitudinal and transverse sonographic evaluation of the anterior hip and groin

Longitudinal

Femoral head and neck, anterior joint recess, iliopsoas muscle, anterior-superior labrum

Transverse

Iliopsoas muscle and tendon, sartorius, tensor fascia lata, direct and indirect tendons of the rectus femoris, femoral head

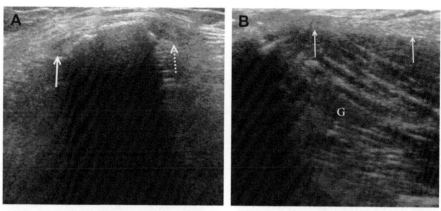

Fig. 3. Transverse (*A*) and longitudinal (*B*) views of the ASIS with the sartorius directed medially (*dashed arrow, A*) and the tensor fascia lata directed laterally (*arrow, A*). The tensor fascia lata tendon is seen longitudinally (*arrows, B*). The gluteus minimus muscle (G) is beneath the tendons.

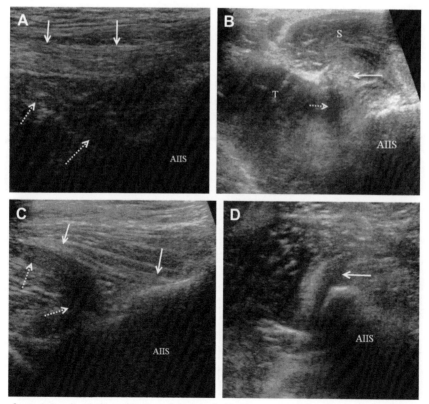

Fig. 4. Rectus femoris tendon in long (*A, C*) and short axis (*B, D*). In *A, B* and *C*, note the direct (*arrows*) and indirect (*dashed arrows*) tendons of the rectus femoris. The indirect tendons in both cases appear hypoechoic because of anisotropy. Note rectus femoris tendon in *D* (*solid arrow*) attaching to the anterior inferior iliac spine (AIIS). S, sartorius; T, tensor fascia lata.

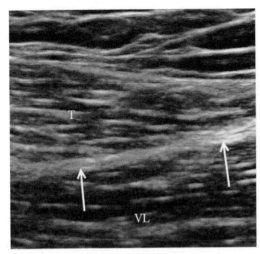

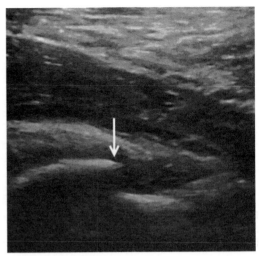

Fig. 5. Tensor fascia lata muscle (T) distally converging into the fascia lata tendon (*arrows*) overlying the vastus lateralis muscle (VL).

Fig. 7. Hip osteoarthrosis. Note spur arising from the femoral head (*arrow*).

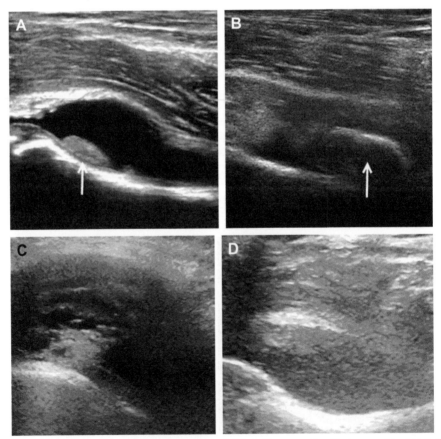

Fig. 6. Spectrum of anterior joint capsule appearances. (*A*) Reactive, aseptic effusion, and incidental echogenic focus of thickened synovium (*arrow*). (*B*) Loose bodies within the joint capsule. (*C*) Synovial proliferation with markedly distended joint capsule and multiple echogenic foci. (*D*) Septic arthritis with distended joint capsule and diffuse internal echoes.

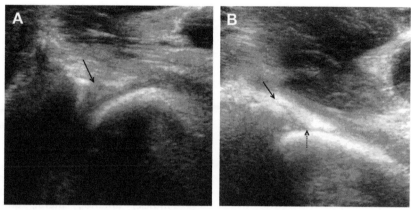

Fig. 8. (*A, B*) Ultrasonographic appearance of anterior-superior labral tear secondary to femoroacetabular impingement. Note the torn labrum with hypoechoic clefts (*arrow*), and decreased distance between the femoral head and torn labrum with the hip in the flexed position (*dashed arrow, B*).

Anterior Hip Evaluation

Structures in the anterior portion of the hip and groin are evaluated in both the long- and short-axis planes (**Figs. 1** and **2**). Scanning in the short axis entails holding the ultrasound probe perpendicular to the long axis of the patient's body. When scanning in the long axis, however, the probe is generally held parallel to the long axis of the femoral neck, such that the resultant images are in a sagittal-oblique plane.[1] This orientation provides good imaging of the femoral head and neck, anterior joint recess, anterior-superior labrum, and the iliopsoas muscle and tendon. Some of these structures are also visible in the transverse plane (**Box 1**).

Other portions of the anterior hip and groin may be added to the evaluation as appropriate for the specific patient symptoms. For example, the sartorius and tensor fascia lata both originate from the anterior-superior iliac spine (ASIS). The sartorius arises from the anterior aspect of the ASIS, and the tensor fascia lata arises from the lateral aspect of the ASIS (**Fig. 3**). The rectus femoris has 3 tendons proximally; the direct tendon

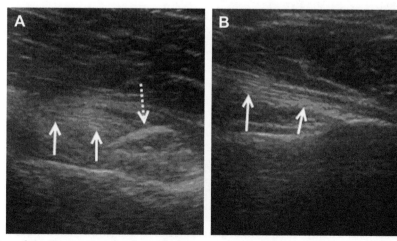

Fig. 9. Avulsion of the iliopsoas tendon from the lesser trochanter (*A*) compared with the normal side (*B*). Note the iliopsoas tendons (*solid arrows*) with avulsed bony fragment (*dashed arrow*) in *A*.

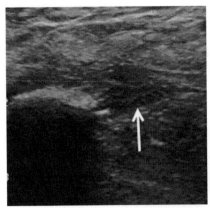

Fig. 10. Tendinosis of the tensor fascia lata. Note thickened, hypoechoic tendon origin (*arrow*).

> **Box 2**
> **Anatomic structures that should be identified during longitudinal and transverse sonographic evaluation of the lateral aspect of the hip**
>
> Longitudinal
>
>   Gluteus medius and minimus muscles and tendons, fascia lata, anterior and lateral trochanteric facets
>
> Transverse
>
>   Gluteus medius and minimus tendons, fascia lata, anterior portion of gluteus maximus muscle, anterior, lateral, and posterior trochanteric facets

originates from the anterior inferior iliac spine, the indirect tendon arises from the superior acetabular ridge, and the reflected tendon extends medially and attaches to the anterior capsule of the hip joint (**Fig. 4**).[1,3] Although these anatomic structures are not universally included in sonographic evaluation of the hip and groin, they should be scanned if tendon abnormality is suspected. The tensor fascia lata is a muscle that tightens the iliotibial tract (**Fig. 5**).

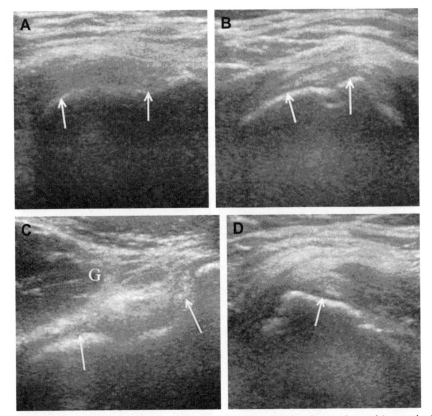

Fig. 11. Longitudinal (*A*) and transverse (*B*) views of gluteus medius tendon (*arrows*) attaching to the lateral facet of the greater trochanter. Longitudinal (*C*) and transverse (*D*) views of the gluteus minimus tendon (*arrows*) attaching to the anterior facet of the greater trochanter. Note the overlying gluteus medius muscle (G).

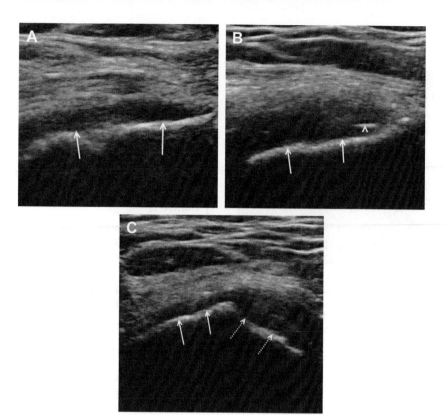

Fig. 12. Longitudinal images of gluteus minimus (*A*) and medius (*B*) tendinosis show thickened, hypoechoic tendons (*arrows*). In *B*, the linear area of hyperechogenicity (*arrowhead*) is evident, suggestive of a partial-thickness intra-substance tear. Transverse view (*C*) shows the gluteus medius (*dashed arrows*) and minimus (*solid arrows*) tendinosis.

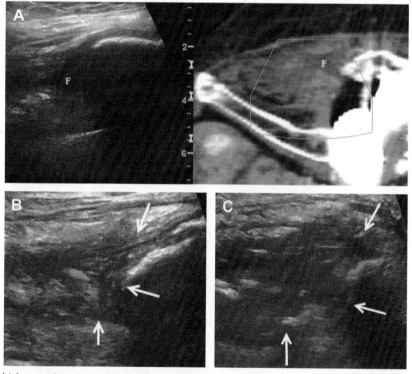

Fig. 13. Full-thickness gluteus medius tendon tear. Coronal ultrasound-CT fusion (*A*) demonstrates fluid (F) around the gluteus medius attachment. No intact tendon is seen. The same findings are seen in additional coronal (*B*) and transverse (*C*) ultrasonographic images (*arrows*).

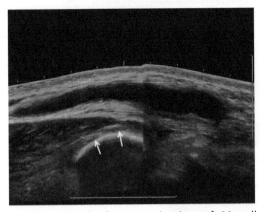

Fig. 14. Longitudinal panoramic view of Morrell-Lavalee lesion represented by a fluid collection immediately deep to the subcutaneous fat, and superficial to the underlying muscle. The gluteus medius tendon is seen attaching to the lateral facet of the greater trochanter (*arrowheads*).

Pathology

Longitudinal evaluation of the anterior hip is the best view for detecting joint effusions (**Fig. 6**). Joint effusions are characteristically anechoic if they represent simple fluid as would be seen in a reactive effusion. Effusions containing internal echoes result from infection and blood products. Loose bodies may also be detected in a joint, which can result from osteoarthritis or, less commonly, osteochondromatosis. There may be synovial proliferation within the joint, which may also result from infection, inflammatory arthritis, pigmented villonodular synovitis, or synovial osteochondromatosis. Imaging characteristics of synovitis include noncompressibility of the distended joint capsule and the presence of color or power Doppler flow in the same region. Synovial proliferation may be hypoechoic, isoechoic, or hyperechoic.[1]

Osteoarthrosis is easily imaged in the anterior portion of the hip joint. Spur formation at the junction between the femoral head and neck is a common finding that can become quite prominent (**Fig. 7**). Osteoarthrosis is sometimes secondary to femoroacetabular impingement, which usually results from a combination of acetabular overgrowth and an aspherical femoral head. In this situation, anterior-superior labral tears are often identified on examination. Sonographic examinations of the hip can be tailored to evaluate for impingement in which dynamic motion of the hip is assessed for contact between the femoral head and acetabulum (**Fig. 8**).

Some of the sports injuries affecting the groin involve the iliopsoas tendon (**Fig. 9**), tensor fascia lata, and rectus femoris tendons, specifically tendinopathy of the tensor fascia lata, and tearing of the rectus femoris tendon. Tensor fascia lata

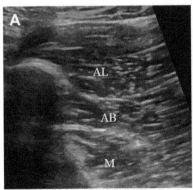
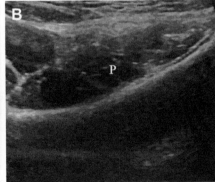

Fig. 15. Normal anatomy of the adductor (*A*) and pectineus musculature (*B*). In *A*, note the adductor longus (AL), adductor brevis (AB), and adductor magnus (M). A transverse view of the pectineus muscle (P) is provided in *B*.

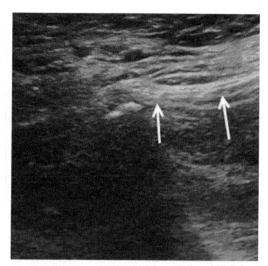

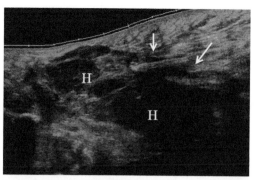

Fig. 17. Panoramic longitudinal view of adductor longus and brevis tendon avulsion with retraction of the adductor longus and brevis (*arrows*). There is significant hypoechoic hematoma formation (H).

Fig. 16. Adductor longus tendon (*arrows*) attaching on the pubis.

tendinopathy (**Fig. 10**) is often seen in sprinters, and presents with pain immediately below the most anterior aspect of the ASIS. Rectus femoris tears most frequently occur in the central aponeurosis, and less commonly the proximal tendon. Iliopsoas tendon avulsion with detachment of the lesser trochanter most commonly occurs in skeletally immature patients, and is caused by activities such as jumping, sprinting, and kicking. If an adult has iliopsoas tendon avulsion, metastatic disease must be considered.[4]

Lateral Hip Evaluation

Lateral evaluation of the hip (**Fig. 11**) concentrates on structures in close proximity to the greater trochanter (**Box 2**). The greater trochanter can be palpated at the level of the pelvis immediately proximal to the femoral shaft. It is composed of 4 facets: anterior, lateral, posterior, and superoposterior. The hip abductors, the gluteus minimus and medius, attach to the greater trochanter. The gluteus minimus tendon attaches to the anterior facet of the greater trochanter. The gluteus medius tendon has an anterior tendon that attaches to the lateral facet, and a posterior tendon that attaches to the superoposterior facet.[1,3,5,6] These tendons can be followed proximally to locate their associated muscles along the lateral aspect of the iliac bone. The gluteus medius muscle is located posterior and superficial to the gluteus minimus muscle. The gluteus maximus muscle overlies the posterior aspect of the gluteus medius tendon. When scanning, a thin, hypoechoic band is found superficial to the gluteus medius and minimus tendons, which represents the fascia lata.[1,2] Both gluteus minimus and medius tendons have an underlying bursa, namely the subgluteus minimus

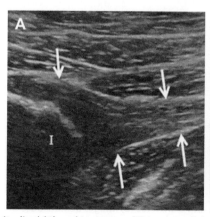

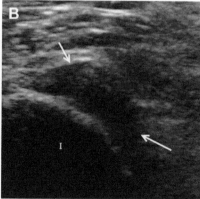

Fig. 18. Longitudinal (*A*) and transverse (*B*) images of the conjoint tendon of the long head of the biceps femoris and semitendinosus (*arrows*) arising from the ischial tuberosity (I).

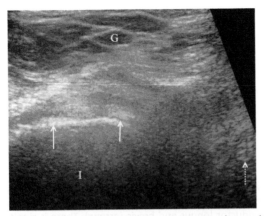

Fig. 19. Transverse image of the conjoint tendon and semimembranosus tendon (*arrows*) arising from the ischial tuberosity (I). The gluteus maximus muscle (G) lies immediately superficial. The sciatic nerve is partially visualized laterally (*dashed arrow*).

> **Box 4**
> **Anatomic structures that should be visualized during evaluation of the posterior aspect of the hip and groin**
>
> Longitudinal
>
>   Hamstring tendon origin, sciatic nerve
>
> Transverse
>
>   Conjoint tendon (biceps femoris and semitendinosus), semimembranosus tendon, sciatic nerve; gluteus maximus, biceps femoris, semitendinosus, semimembranosus muscles

bursa and the subgluteus medius bursa. The trochanteric bursa is a third bursa, closely associated with the greater trochanter, which can be found along the posterior and lateral trochanteric facets.[2,5,6] None of these bursae are normally visible.

Pathology
As with other tendons, the gluteus medius and minimus tendons are prone to tendinosis and tearing. Tears are especially common in the gluteus medius tendon. The most common patient demographics include women in late middle age and patients who have had steroid injections or total hip arthroplasties.[2,3,7] Tears of these tendons can be partial (**Fig. 12**) or complete (**Fig. 13**), and

have imaging characteristics of tendon tears elsewhere in the body. Trochanteric bursitis can also occur, in which the bursa becomes distended with fluid.

Morrell-Lavalee lesions (**Fig. 14**) are very common, and are characteristically found in the proximal thigh and near the greater trochanter. These lesions develop as the result of trauma, and are described as closed degloving injuries. On imaging, they are represented by fluid collections between the subcutaneous fat and the underlying fascia.[1,3,8]

Medial Compartment Evaluation

The medial portion of the hip is best evaluated with the patient's knee bent and hip abducted and externally rotated. The structures in this region include the adductor musculature, located just lateral to the pubic symphysis (**Box 3**). From superficial to deep, these muscles include the

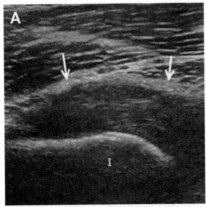
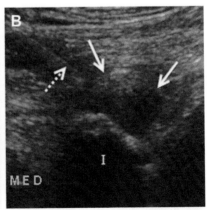

Fig. 20. Proximal hamstring tendinosis. Longitudinal (*A*), and transverse (*B*) images demonstrate thickened, hypoechoic hamstring tendons (*arrows*) originating from the ischial tuberosity (I). Note the needle in the upper left-hand corner (*dashed arrow, B*).

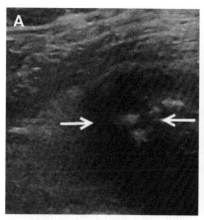
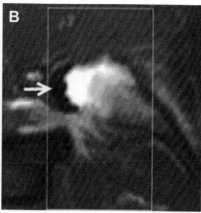

Fig. 21. Ultrasound (*A*) and MR (*B*) images of a high-grade partial hamstring tear involving the conjoint and semi-membranosus tendons (*arrows*).

adductor longus, adductor brevis, and adductor magnus (**Figs. 15** and **16**). These muscles are usually visualized transversely with the ultrasound probe held in a plane along the long axis of the patient's femur; however, they may also be seen longitudinally as they insert on the pubis. The pectineus (see **Fig. 15B**) and gracilis muscles can also be evaluated if desired.

Pathology

One of the most common hip and groin injuries that occur medially is tear or avulsion of the adductor musculature (**Fig. 17**). This injury most commonly involves the adductor longus, and is characteristically seen in athletes. Imaging features of these injuries include tendon retraction and hematoma formation.

Posterior Hip and Groin Evaluation

The conjoint tendon of the long head of the biceps femoris and semitendinosus and the semimembranosus tendon both originate from the lateral aspect of the ischial tuberosity (**Fig. 18**). At its most proximal extent, the semimembranosus tendon is lateral to the conjoint tendon. Following the tendons distally from their origin, the conjoint tendon becomes superficial and lateral to the semimembranosus tendon. The sciatic nerve is also found in this region, lateral to the origin of the hamstring tendons (**Fig. 19**). These structures are scanned in both the longitudinal and transverse planes with the ischial tuberosity as a landmark (**Box 4**).

Pathology

Hamstring tendinosis (**Fig. 20**) occurs as the result of chronic microtrauma. Hamstring injuries are usually secondary to participation in sports

such as soccer and water skiing, although patients in other demographic groups are often affected. Tears may be located within the tendon substance or more distally at the myotendinous junction. Sonographic assessment is difficult because of the proximity of the adjacent bones and patient discomfort with transducer pressure. Avulsed bone fragments may accompany tendon ruptures, and surrounding hematoma formation (**Figs. 21** and **22**) may also be present. Assessment of the ischial tuberosity is important. As with other locations, partial and complete tears may be accompanied by significant bony irregularity.[1]

GROIN HERNIAS
Introduction

Ultrasonography can used to evaluate groin hernias. The reasons that give sonography advantages over other imaging modalities in assessment of sports injuries are also true in the detection and characterization of hernias. Similar equipment is used (**Fig. 23**).

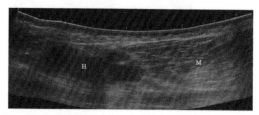

Fig. 22. Full-thickness tear of the proximal conjoint tendon of the biceps femoris and semitendinosus with hypoechoic hematoma (H). The muscles are seen distally (M).

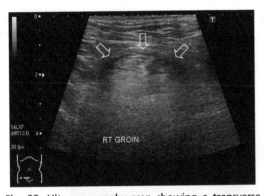

RT GROIN

Fig. 23. Ultrasonography scan showing a transverse section of the right groin. The image has been optimized to demonstrate the relevant anatomy. An adequate depth has been selected to show the deep structures and possible origin of the inguinal hernia (*open arrows*). The focal zone has been set to the desired region of interest. The frequency of insonation, dynamic range, and contrast map have been optimized for a superficial musculoskeletal structure. Note the use of a high frame rate (more than 16 frames per second). With some equipment, it is possible to sweep the insonating beam and create a wider field of view with a linear transducer, which has the advantage of making it easier to appreciate the anatomy of the groin.

Sonographic evaluation of the groin hernia is not part of routine evaluation.[9] When it is systematically performed, it can result in an accurate diagnosis and provide useful information for treatment.[10] The first step is to communicate with the patient about the presenting symptoms, for example, pain, mass, and when the symptoms are most consistently reproduced. This evaluation can help guide the dynamic maneuvers to be performed.

Using the pubic symphysis as a landmark, scanning is performed by searching from the medial to lateral position for an abnormal mass or change in the anatomy. The patient can be asked to cough or perform a Valsalva maneuver. The patient should also be scanned in the upright position. This section describes the anatomy of the groin and serves to acquaint the reader with the normal and abnormal sonographic findings in adult inguinal hernias.

Anatomy

Abdominal hernias are usually inguinal (75%) and are more common in males than females (M/F 8:1). Less common sites include the femoral (15%) and umbilical hernia (8%).[11] Women are more likely than men to have femoral hernias. The inguinal hernia is a protrusion of the abdominal cavity contents through an aperture or weakness of the abdominal wall. Inguinal hernias are one of the most common reasons for emergency surgery in patients older than 50 years and the second most common reason for surgery after acute appendicitis in Europe and the United States. In the newborn, a patent processus vaginalis is the cause of the inguinal hernia. In adults and elderly, wall stress and weakness of the abdominal wall, respectively, are responsible for the inguinal hernias.

Although inguinal hernias are traditionally diagnosed by physical examination, there are limitations when the symptoms are vague or the signs are indeterminate.[11–13] Factors that can mask the signs of a hernia include obesity, a small hernia, or previous surgery. The groin region may be divided into the inguinal canal and the femoral triangle.[14] The canal is a tube formed by the medial free edge of the external oblique anastomosis (the inguinal ligament) curling back onto itself. It is U-shaped in cross section.

In males, the spermatic cord runs through the canal. The cord enters via the deep inguinal ring (which lies lateral to the inferior epigastric artery,

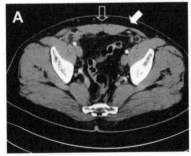
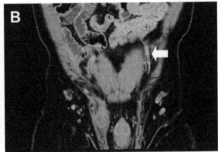

Fig. 24. Transverse section (*A*) and coronal reconstruction (*B*) from a CT scan through the pelvis. The linea alba is seen in the midline between the bellies of the rectus abdominis muscle (*open arrow*). Moving laterally, the inferior epigastric vessels (artery and veins) can be identified as running just medial to the linea semilunaris and deep the lateral margin of the belly of the rectus abdominis muscle (*white arrow*).

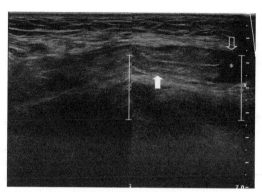

Fig. 25. Ultrasonography scan showing a longitudinal section of a direct inguinal hernia that has entered into the scrotum. Note the hernia sac is a thin echogenic line that often merges with the adjacent soft tissue (*open arrow*). A small amount of fluid is seen at the tip of the sac (*asterisk*). Bowel loops are present within the sac (*white arrow*) and prolonged observation may show peristalsis of the bowel.

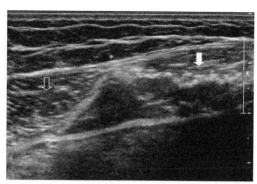

Fig. 27. Ultrasonography scan showing a transverse section of the left groin. A mesh (*white arrow*) has been placed over the left deep inguinal ring. The belly of the rectus abdominis can be seen medially (*open arrow*) while the oblique muscles of the abdomen are seen laterally. The linea semilunaris (*asterisk*) is a useful landmark.

halfway along the posterior wall of the inguinal canal), runs through the canal, and exits via the superficial inguinal ring (superior and medial to the pubic tubercle). The spermatic cord is surrounded by the fascial layers derived from the abdominal wall muscles. It contains the ductus deferens and its artery, testicular artery and pampiniform (venous) plexus, genital branch of the genitofemoral nerve, lymphatic vessels and sympathetic nerve fibers, fat, and connective tissues.

The ilioinguinal nerve runs along the front of the cord.

In females, the inguinal canal contains the round ligament of uterus. As a result, the canal is much smaller in women.

Imaging Protocol

A systematic approach to imaging the groin is helpful to ensure that all relevant information is acquired. A useful starting point is the midline of the anterior abdominal wall at the position of the linea alba (**Fig. 24**A). With a linear transducer in a transverse position, image optimization is performed to ensure adequate depth of view and

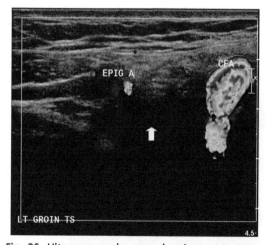

Fig. 26. Ultrasonography scan showing a transverse section of the left groin. Note that the hernia (*white arrow*) lies between the left inferior epigastric artery (EPIG A) and left common femoral artery (CFA), indicating that this is an indirect hernia. A direct hernia would be seen medial to the inferior epigastric artery (see **Fig. 7**).

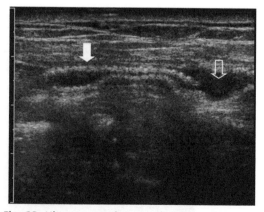

Fig. 28. Ultrasonography scan showing a transverse section of the right groin. A mesh (*white arrow*) has been placed over the deep inguinal ring. A small amount of fluid is seen next the mesh (*open arrow*) that usually resolves spontaneously.

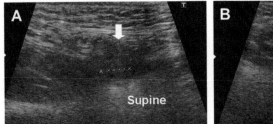
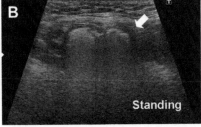

Fig. 29. (A, B) Ultrasonography scan showing a transverse section of the right groin. There is a direct inguinal hernia (*white arrow*) that becomes obvious when the patient stands upright. The neck of the hernia is marked with a caliper in the supine image. Note the echogenic shadowing caused by air in the herniated bowel loops.

use of focusing to see the details needed. Moving inferiorly and laterally, the inferior epigastric vessels can be identified as posterior to the belly of the rectus abdominis (see **Fig. 24**B). By correlating with the bony landmarks of the pubic tubercle and the anterior-superior iliac spine, the inguinal canal can be easily identified. It is usually parallel to the skin crease, but obesity and soft-tissue laxity can result in variation in the usual surface anatomy. By turning the transducer to an oblique position, the inguinal canal can be seen parallel to the transducer in a longitudinal axis. The transducer can also be rotated so that it is orthogonal to the inguinal canal that is seen on a short-axis view.

Although the patient is usually scanned in a supine position initially, the patient should also be examined in the upright position. Soft-tissue displacement can make this challenging in an obese patient, but reducible hernias are often

best seen with this maneuver. Provocative tests such as coughing (Videos 1 and 2) and the Valsalva maneuver help to elucidate the contents of a hernia sac (Video 3).

Imaging Findings

An inguinal hernia is recognized as a mass arising from the inguinal canal. The sonographic appearance depends on the soft tissue that has herniated from the abdominal cavity. In the majority of cases, this will be omental and mesenteric fat or bowel loops. It should be noted that the differential diagnoses include rare lesions such as endometriosis of the round ligament,[15] round ligament varicosities,[16] mesothelial cyst,[17] and hydrocele of the canal of Nuck.[18] Other groin masses that are more common include enlarged reactive lymph nodes and posttraumatic pseudoaneurysm. The history from the patient and

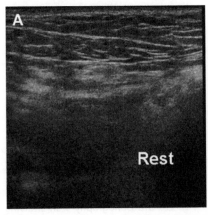
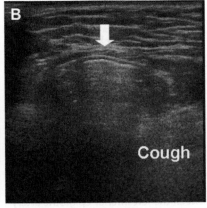

Fig. 30. (A, B) Ultrasonography scan showing a transverse section of the right groin. There is a direct inguinal hernia (*white arrow*) that becomes obvious when the patient is asked to cough. Other actions that raise the intra-abdominal pressure (eg, a Valsalva maneuver) may be used. The advantages of asking the patient to cough are ease of instruction and compliance.

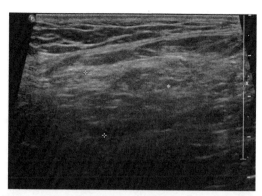

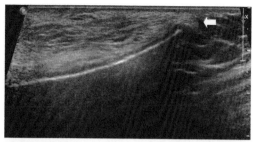

Fig. 32. Ultrasonography scan showing a longitudinal section of a superficial groin lipoma that arises from the subcutaneous fat. Although this lesion lacks a positive cough impulse, the superior border of the lesion can be identified by palpation and sonographically (*white arrow*).

Fig. 31. Ultrasonography scan showing a longitudinal section of a direct inguinal hernia (*asterisk*) that has entered into the scrotum. This section consisted of mesenteric fat, and no movement was detected when the patient was asked to cough or perform a Valsalva maneuver. However, the superior end of the groin mass could not be identified, and the contents of the hernia could be traced to the superficial inguinal ring.

difficult to detect but can usually be found (**Figs. 27** and **28**).[19]

physical findings are usually sufficient to make a diagnosis.

Diagnostic Criteria

An inguinal hernia can be confidently diagnosed if there are bowel loops demonstrated in a sac arising from the inguinal canal (**Fig. 25**). The presence of peristalsis is considered pathognomonic (Video 4). It should be noted that other abdominal contents (eg, fat) can be found in the hernia sac as well. The relationship of the neck of the hernia sac to the inferior epigastric artery is critical to differentiating an indirect from a direct hernia (**Fig. 26**).

These criteria are also applicable to the postoperative patient (Video 5). The use of mesh is more common in surgery today. Mesh can be

Pearls, Pitfalls, and Variants

A reducible hernia may not be obvious in the supine position. Standing a patient upright can make an inguinal hernia appear (**Fig. 29**). Other maneuvers that increase intra-abdominal pressure include asking the patient to cough (**Fig. 30**) or perform a Valsalva maneuver.

An irreducible hernia may not be recognized if there is no cough impulse detected (**Fig. 31**). The inability to get above the lesion as it ascends in the inguinal canal is helpful in deciding the origin of a groin mass (**Fig. 32**).

A small hernia may be missed, especially if it is reducible (Video 6); this can be avoided by a systematic search in the groin covering the entire inguinal ligament. Review of cine clips with a fast frame rate (more than 16 frames per second) is usually helpful in documenting small transient hernias (**Fig. 33**).

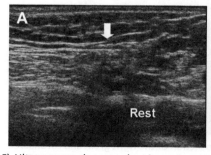

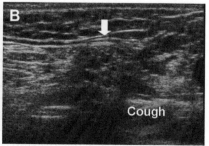

Fig. 33. (*A, B*) Ultrasonography scan showing a transverse section of the right groin. There is a small inguinal hernia (*white arrow*) that becomes obvious when the patient is asked to cough. However, the findings are transient and the use of a cine clip is recommended for documentation.

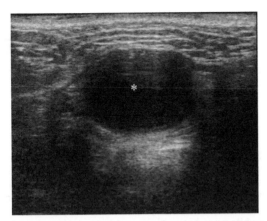

Fig. 34. Ultrasonography scan showing a transverse section of the right groin. A small seroma (*asterisk*) that is almost anechoic is seen; this is palpable because of its superficial location. The fluid in a seroma may have some echoes and be hypoechoic, but it is generally unilocular with a bland appearance.

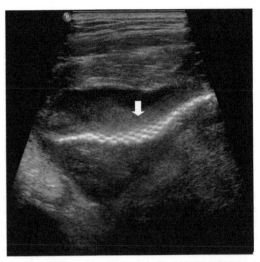

Fig. 36. Ultrasonography scan showing a transverse section of the right groin, showing the mesh (*white arrow*) used in a laparoscopic inguinal hernia repair displaced by a large postoperative hematoma. Note the woven appearance of the mesh as it is passes obliquely through the insonating ultrasound beam.

In the postoperative patient with pain or a mass, recurrence of the hernia should be suspected. Alternative diagnoses include a seroma (**Fig. 34**) or hematoma (**Fig. 35**). In the case of a large hematoma, the mesh can be displaced (**Fig. 36**).

Pathology

Most asymptomatic inguinal hernias can be safely managed without surgery. However, over time most patients will develop symptoms. The most common is pain, and the patients will require surgery.[20] Acute complications such as strangulation, intestinal obstruction, and infarction are uncommon but can be life threatening.

What the Referring Physician Needs to Know

Imaging is seldom required in the evaluation of the patient with an inguinal hernia. When performed, it can be extremely useful in the differentiation of the direct from the indirect inguinal hernia. Diagnostic pitfalls can occur with the easily reducible hernia, small hernia, and rare differential diagnoses for a groin mass. Additional imaging, when needed, may include CT or MR scans.

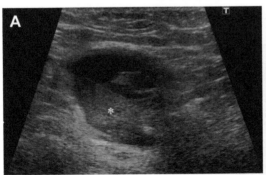
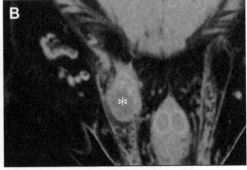

Fig. 35. (*A, B*) Ultrasonography scan showing a transverse section of the right groin and coronal reconstruction of the right groin from a contemporaneous CT scan. A small hematoma (*asterisk*) that consists of a mixture of solid and fluid is seen; this is palpable because of its superficial location. Unlike the seroma, a hematoma usually has a complex appearance on sonography. Note the greater detail seen with the ultrasonography scan.

SUMMARY

Imaging of the groin can be performed with ultrasound. The superior spatial resolution and ability to perform dynamic maneuvers make it an excellent first choice as an imaging modality. When dealing with sports injuries, the ability to detect soft-tissue lesions rapidly allows appropriate therapy or return to activity. In the evaluation of hernias, the ability to detect symptomatic but clinically occult hernias is an advantage that can aid in the treatment of patients.

SUPPLEMENTARY DATA

Videos related to this article can be found online at doi:http://dx.doi.org/10.1016/j.cult.2012.08.002.

REFERENCES

1. Jacobson JA. Fundamentals of musculoskeletal ultrasound 2007.
2. Bianchi S, Poletti P, Martinoli C, et al. Ultrasound appearance of tendon tears. Part 2: lower extremity and myotendinous tears. Skeletal Radiol 2006;35:63–77.
3. Bianchi S, Martinoli C. Ultrasound of the musculoskeletal system 2007.
4. Bancroft LW, Blankenbaker DG. Imaging of the tendons about the pelvis. Am J Roentgenol 2010;195:605–17.
5. Connell DA, Bass C, Sykes CJ, et al. Sonographic evaluation of gluteus medius and minimus tendinopathy. Eur J Radiol 2003;13:1339–47.
6. Pfirrmann CW, Chung CB, Theuman NH, et al. Greater trochanter of the hip: attachment of the abductor mechanism and a complex of three bursae—MR imaging and MR bursography in cadavers and MR imaging in asymptomatic volunteers. Radiology 2001;221:469–77.
7. Kong A, Van der Vliet A, Zadow S. MRI and US of gluteal tendinopathy in greater trochanteric pain syndrome. Eur J Radiol 2007;17:1772–83.
8. Mellado JM, Perez del Palomar L, Diaz L, et al. Long-standing Morel-Lavalee lesions of the trochanteric region and proximal thigh: MRI features in five patients. AJR Am J Roentgenol 2004;182:1289–94.
9. Rosenberg J, Bisgaard T, Kehlet H, et al, Danish Hernia Database. Danish Hernia Database recommendations for the management of inguinal and femoral hernia in adults. Dan Med Bull 2011;58(2):C4243.
10. Light D, Ratnasingham K, Banerjee A, et al. The role of ultrasound scan in the diagnosis of occult inguinal hernias. Int J Surg 2011;9(2):169–72.
11. Lassandro F, Iasiello F, Pizza NL, et al. Abdominal hernias: radiological features. World J Gastrointest Endosc 2011;3(6):110–7.
12. Grant T, Neuschler E, Hartz W 3rd. Groin pain in women: use of sonography to detect occult hernias. J Ultrasound Med 2011;30(12):1701–7.
13. Jamadar DA, Jacobson JA, Morag Y, et al. Sonography of inguinal region hernias. Am J Roentgenol 2006;187(1):185–90.
14. Shadbolt CL, Heinze SB, Dietrich RB. Imaging of groin masses: inguinal anatomy and pathologic conditions revisited. Radiographics 2001;21(Spec No):S261–71.
15. Calò PG, Esu F, Tatti A, et al. Isolated inguinal endometriosis. Case report with ultrasonographic preoperative diagnosis. G Chir 2011;32(5):263–5.
16. Kahriman G, Donmez H, Mavili E, et al. Bilateral round ligament varicosities mimicking an inguinal hernia in pregnancy: case report. J Clin Ultrasound 2010;38(9):512–4.
17. Aarabi S, Drugas G, Avansino JR. Mesothelial cyst presenting as an irreducible inguinal mass. J Pediatr Surg 2010;45(6):e19–21.
18. Caviezel A, Montet X, Schwartz J, et al. Female hydrocele: the cyst of Nuck. Urol Int 2009;82(2):242–5.
19. Jamadar DA, Jacobson JA, Girish G, et al. Abdominal wall hernia mesh repair: sonography of mesh and common complications. J Ultrasound Med 2008;27(6):907–17.
20. Mizrahi H, Parker MC. Management of asymptomatic inguinal hernia: a systematic review of the evidence. Arch Surg 2012;147(3):277–81.

Ultrasound of the Knee

Joseph G. Craig, MB ChB[a,b],*, David Fessell, MD[c]

KEYWORDS

- Ultrasound • Knee • Normal ultrasound anatomy knee • Quadriceps tendon • Patellar tendon
- Baker cyst • Knee joint effusion

KEY POINTS

- Advanced imaging of the knee joint is most commonly performed using MR imaging.
- Ultrasound can display much of the normal knee anatomy but has major limitations in assessing the meniscus and cruciate ligaments and cannot image through cortex/subchondral bone.
- In evaluation of knee joint effusion and ultrasound-guided aspiration, ultrasound is unsurpassed.
- Ultrasound is very useful in the clinical setting of rupture of the quadriceps tendon or patellar tendon and in the assessment and rupture of Baker cysts.

INTRODUCTION

This article reviews the ultrasound appearance of normal knee anatomy and of common knee pathology.

TECHNIQUE

In ultrasound evaluation of the knee, most commonly a 5- to 12-mHz general purpose transducer is used in the axial, coronal, and sagittal planes, depending on anatomy and pathology. The knee should be scanned in a systematic fashion. Having the knee in slight flexion, supported by a rolled up towel or a cushion, is useful for evaluation of the anterior structures, because tension is placed on the extensor mechanism.

NORMAL ANATOMY
Anterior Structures

It is easiest to begin ultrasound evaluation anteriorly by scanning the quadriceps tendon and patellar tendon.

Quadriceps tendon

The quadriceps tendon is formed from aponeurotic tendinous contributions by the rectus femoris, vastus medialis, intermedius, and lateralis muscles.[1] The quadriceps tendon inserts onto the superior pole of the patella. The tendon is scanned in the longitudinal and transverse planes (**Fig. 1**). The tendon can be easily followed from the musculotendinous junction of the quadriceps to the superior pole of the patella. The normal tendon has a hyperechoic, fibrillar appearance (see **Fig. 1**B, C). Immediately deep to the tendon is the suprapatellar bursa and suprapatellar fat pad (see **Fig. 1**B).

Patellar tendon

This tendon is scanned in longitudinal and transverse planes. It starts at the inferior pole of the patella and courses inferiorly to the tibial tuberosity. The tendon has a compact fibrillar appearance, with Hoffa's fat pad immediately deep to the tendon (**Fig. 2**).

Lateral Knee

The normal anatomy of the lateral knee is seen in **Fig. 3**.

Iliotibial band

The iliotibial band is a longitudinal fibrous reinforcement of the fascia lata. The iliotibial band runs down the anterolateral aspect of the knee to

[a] Department of Radiology, Henry Ford Hospital, 2799 West Grad Bonlevovd, Detroit, MI 48202, USA; [b] Wayne State University Medical School, 540 East Canfield, Detroit, MI 48201, USA; [c] University of Michigan Medical School, 1301 Catherine Road, Ann Arbor, MI 48109, USA
* Corresponding author. Wayne State University Medical School, 540 East Canfield, Detroit, MI 48201.
E-mail address: josephc@rad.hfh.edu

Ultrasound Clin 7 (2012) 475–486
http://dx.doi.org/10.1016/j.cult.2012.08.003
1556-858X/12/$ – see front matter © 2012 Published by Elsevier Inc.

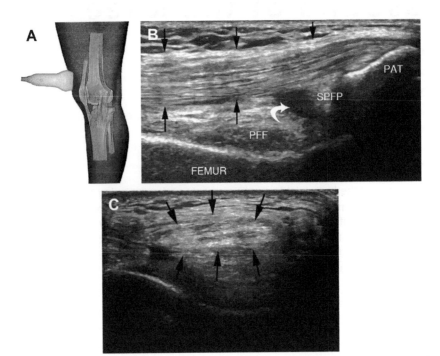

Fig. 1. Normal quadriceps tendon. (A) Normal positioning of the transducer for the longitudinal view of the quadriceps tendon. (B) Normal longitudinal view of the quadriceps tendon (*black arrows*) attaching to the patella. Notice there is a small amount of fluid in the suprapatellar bursa (*curved arrow*). PFF, prefemoral fat; SPFP, suprapatellar fat pad; PAT, patella. (C) Normal transverse view of the quadriceps tendon (*arrows*). Note the hyperechoic appearance of the tendon.

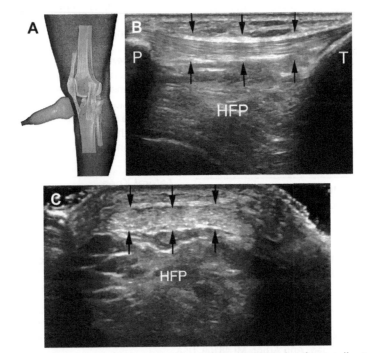

Fig. 2. Normal patellar tendon. (A) Normal positioning of the transducer for the patellar tendon. (B) Normal longitudinal view of the patellar tendon (*arrows*). Note the normal hyperechoic appearance of the tendon. HFP, Hoffa's fat pad; P, patella; T, tibial tuberosity. (C) Normal axial view of the patellar tendon (*arrows*). Again note the normal hyperechoic appearance of the tendon. HFP, Hoffa's fat pad.

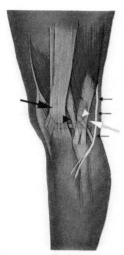

Fig. 3. Normal anatomy of the lateral knee. Note the iliotibial band (*black arrow*), popliteus tendon (*white arrowhead*), fibular collateral ligament (*black arrowhead*), distal biceps tendon (*white arrow*), and common peroneal nerve (*short black arrows*).

insert on Gerdy tubercle at the anterolateral aspect of the tibia. The iliotibial band is easily identified on ultrasound and can be followed from the lateral thigh to the tubercle (**Fig. 4**). It courses adjacent to the anterior aspect of the lateral femoral condyle.

Popliteus tendon
The popliteus tendon courses along the posterolateral aspect of the tibia, adjacent to the posterior aspect of the posterior horn of the lateral meniscus, and curves to course anteriorly and superiorly to insert into the notch in the lateral femoral condyle. The notch for the popliteus is easily identified during ultrasound examination by

scanning just posterior to the iliotibial band in the coronal plane (**Fig. 5**A). The popliteus tendon in identified as a hyperechoic fibrillar structure (see **Fig. 5**B).

Fibular collateral ligament
The fibular collateral ligament (FCL), round and cordlike, runs in an oblique paracoronal plane from the lateral epicondyle of the femur just above the notch for the popliteus inferiorly and posteriorly to insert on the lateral aspect of the fibular head (**Fig. 6**). The distal extent is covered by the biceps femoris tendon.[1] It can be challenging to image the entire extent of the FCL in one plane because of its slightly oblique course. Anisotropy may be seen at the proximal or distal aspect of the ligament (see **Fig. 6**B, C). The distal ligament forms the lateral boundary of the popliteal fossa.[1] It courses distally to the head of the fibula and has lesser contributions to the lateral condyle of the tibia and the adjacent fascia.[1]

Biceps femoris tendon
The biceps femoris tendon courses slightly obliquely in the coronal plane to insert on the lateral aspect of the fibula. The tendon typically has a hyperechoic, fibrillar appearance (**Fig. 7**).

Common peroneal nerve
The common peroneal nerve (L4–S2) courses on the posterolateral aspect of the knee joint, posterior to the biceps femoris tendon. The nerve appears cord-like on coronal sections and is round in axial sections. It can be followed from the bifurcation of the sciatic nerve in the superior popliteal fossa inferiorly and laterally to the level of the fibular neck (**Fig. 8**). It crosses the lateral head of the gastrocnemius and winds around the posterior aspect of the neck of the fibula and divides into superficial and deep branches.

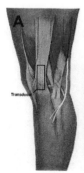
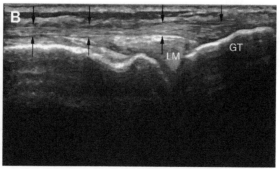

Fig. 4. Iliotibial band. (*A*) Positioning of the transducer for imaging the iliotibial band. (*B*) Normal longitudinal view of the iliotibial band (*arrows*). LM, anterior horn lateral meniscus, GT, Gerdy tubercle.

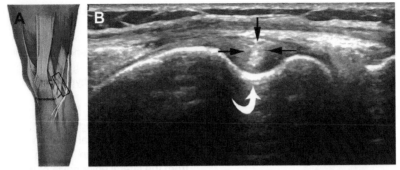

Fig. 5. Popliteus tendon. (*A*) Normal positioning of the transducer for the popliteus tendon. (*B*) Popliteus tendon (*black arrows*) inserting into the notch for the popliteus (*curved arrow*).

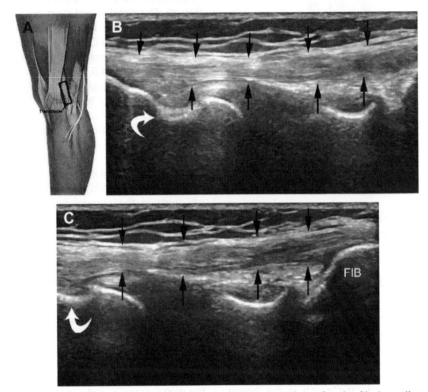

Fig. 6. Fibular collateral ligament. (*A*) Normal positioning of the transducer for the fibular collateral ligament. (*B, C*) Normal longitudinal image of the fibular collateral ligament (*black arrows*). Note it is often difficult to image the entire ligament on one view because of anisotropy. In (*B*), the distal portion of the ligament is not visualized. Note the origin of the ligament from just above the notch for the popliteus (*white curved arrow*). Fib, fibular head.

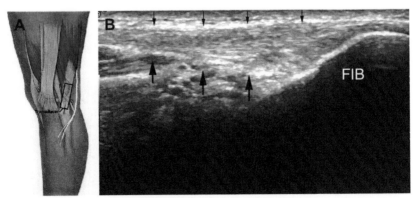

Fig. 7. Distal biceps femoris tendon. (*A*) Normal positioning of the transducer for the distal biceps femoris tendon. (*B*) Normal distal biceps femoris tendon (*black arrows*) inserting onto the fibular head. Note the normal hyperechoic appearance of the tendon. Fib, fibular head.

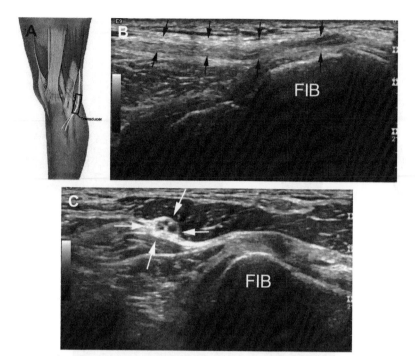

Fig. 8. Common peroneal nerve. (*A*) Normal positioning of the transducer for the common peroneal nerve. (*B*) Normal longitudinal appearance of the cord-like common peroneal nerve (*arrows*). The nerve courses around the fibular neck and then divides. Fib, fibular head. (*C*) Normal axial oval appearance of the common peroneal nerve (*arrows*). Fib, fibular head.

Posterior Knee

The popliteal neurovascular bundle is easily identified on both axial and coronal sections. The medial head of gastrocnemius/semimembranosus interface is best identified on axial sections and are crucial landmarks for identifying a Baker cyst (**Fig. 9**). (See further discussion in later section on Baker cyst.)

Medial Knee

Medial collateral ligament

The medial collateral ligament (MCL) is a flat, quadrilateral ligament arising from the medial femoral condyle and attaching to the tibia. It is best seen in the coronal plane (**Fig. 10A–D**). The MCL has a superficial and deep layer. On ultrasound, the superficial and deep layers frequently

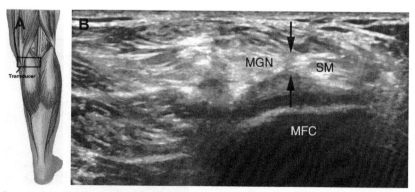

Fig. 9. Normal posteromedial knee. (*A*) Positioning of the transducer for the posteromedial knee. (*B*) Transverse image through the posteromedial knee shows the normal medial head of gastrocnemius (MGN) and semimembranosus tendons (SM). Note the interface between the tendons (*arrows*). No evidence of a Baker cyst is seen.

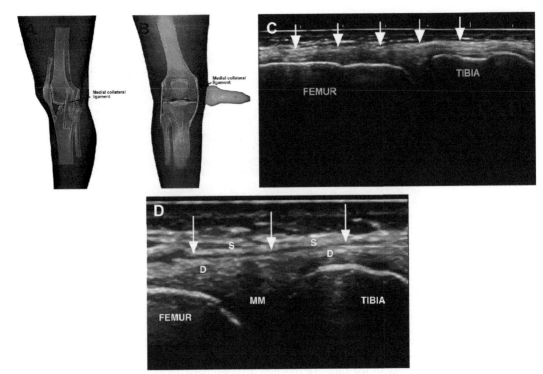

Fig. 10. Medial collateral ligament. (*A*) Normal medial collateral ligament. Sagittal view of the normal medial collateral ligament of the knee. (*B*) Positioning of the transducer. (*C*) Normal ultrasound appearance. Note the hyperechoic appearance of the ligament (*arrows*) attaching to the femur and tibia. (*D*) Coned-down view of the medial collateral ligament showing the trilaminar appearance. Note the hypoechoic slit (*arrows*) between the superficial (*S*) and deep (*D*) parts of the ligament representing either a bursa or fibrofatty tissue. MM, medial meniscus. (*From* Craig JG. Ultrasound of ligaments and bone. Ultrasound Clin 2007;2(4):627.)

can be distinguished. Both layers are hyperechoic. A small hypoechoic linear area between the layers represents either fibrofatty tissue or a potential bursa (see **Fig. 10**D). The width of the normal MCL, adjacent to the concavity of the medial surface of the medial femoral condyle, is 3 to 6 mm.[2]

Pes anserine tendons

The pes anserine tendons comprise the common insertion of the sartorius, semitendinosus, and gracilis onto the anteromedial tibia. The common tendon is best identified in coronal and axial planes anterior and inferior to the tibial attachment of the medial collateral ligament (**Fig. 11**).

PATHOLOGY
Rupture of the Quadriceps and Patellar Tendons

Rupture of the quadriceps tendon is more likely to occur in older patients and those with systemic disease, including diabetes mellitus, chronic renal

failure, gout, and hyperparathyroidism.[3] As with all ultrasound examinations, radiographs, if available, should be carefully reviewed before sonography is performed (**Fig. 12**A). The patella may also be low-lying in some cases of quadriceps rupture. Care should also be taken to review the suprapatellar region for any possible bone fragments, which

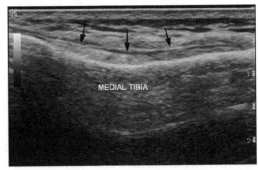

Fig. 11. Normal pes anserine tendon insertion (*arrows*).

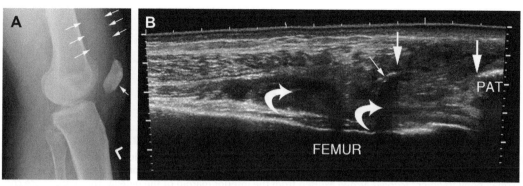

Fig. 12. Quadriceps tendon tear. (*A*) Lateral radiograph of the knee shows a low-lying patella (*short arrow*). Notice the suprapatellar soft tissue swelling and a large knee joint effusion (*long arrows*). (*B*) Longitudinal view of the quadriceps tendon shows discontinuity and retraction of tendon (*long arrows*) with a large complex suprapatellar effusion (*curved arrows*). Contrast the appearance with the normal tendon as shown in **Fig. 1**B. Note also the small fragment of avulsed bone (*short arrow*), not seen in the radiograph. PAT, patella.

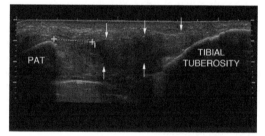

Fig. 13. Acute rupture of the patellar tendon. Longitudinal image shows a proximal tear (calipers) of the patellar tendon. Note the redundancy and bunching up of the distal tendon (*arrows*). PAT, patella.

may represent from the superior patella. Full-thickness, full-width tear results in complete discontinuity of the tendon (see **Fig. 12**B). As in evaluation of the rotator cuff, tears may be full thickness and less-than-full width. How much of the tendon is torn and the degree of retraction are important to document.

Rupture of the patellar tendon is more likely to occur in younger patients, particularly children and adolescents.[3] After rupture, the patella may be high-riding. Ultrasound examination can reveal complete or partial discontinuity of the tendon (**Figs. 13** and **14**).

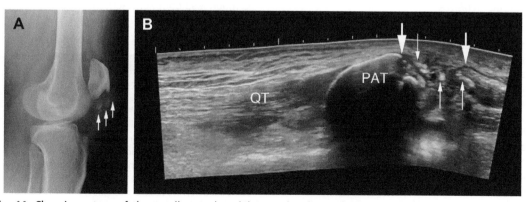

Fig. 14. Chronic rupture of the patellar tendon. (*A*) Lateral radiograph shows well-formed ossific fragments (*arrows*) inferior to the patella. (*B*) Longitudinal extended field of view image shows discontinuity of the proximal patellar tendon (*large arrows*) and small linear foci (*thin arrows*) representing osseous fragments. Note the retraction and discontinuity of the tendon when compared with the normal patellar tendon in **Fig. 2**B. QT, quadriceps tendon; PAT, patella.

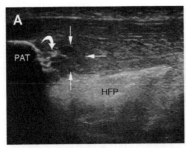
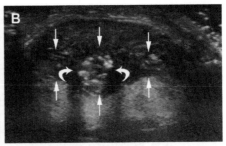

Fig. 15. Jumper's knee. (A) Longitudinal image through the proximal patellar tendon shows diffuse swelling and hypoechogenicity of the proximal tendon particularly affecting the deeper tendon (*straight arrows*). Note also the small bony fragment (*curved arrow*) avulsed from the inferior margin of the patella. The changes are consistent with patellar tendonosis (Jumper's knee). HFP, Hoffa's fat pad; PAT, patella. (B) Transverse image through the proximal patellar tendon. Note the diffuse swelling of the deep portion of the middle third of the patellar tendon (*straight arrows*). Note also the hyperechoic area (*curved arrows*) representing the small avulsed osseous fragments.

Jumper's Knee

Jumper's knee occurs from chronic traction on the inferior pole of the patella and is usually seen in adolescents and young adults. In children, the condition is referred to as Sinding-Larsen-Johansson disease. Patients usually have a history of participation in a sporting activity, most commonly basketball or running. On ultrasound examination, changes are most commonly seen immediately adjacent to the inferior pole of the patella, involving the deep fibers in the middle third or medial third of the tendon (**Fig. 15**). Color imaging may show hyperemia. Typical changes are loss of the normal fibrillar pattern of the tendon, with hypoechogenicity and swelling of the proximal tendon. The area may be tender on ultrasound examination. Small hyperechogenic structures may represent slivers of bone or areas of posttraumatic ossification.

Osgood-Schlatter

Chronic traction on the inferior patellar tendon at the attachment to the tibial tuberosity can be associated with an ossicle at the tibial tuberosity and is referred to as Osgood-Schlatter disease. The condition is primarily a clinical diagnosis, but occasionally imaging is requested. Ultrasound examination will show soft tissue swelling over the tibial tuberosity, thickening of the distal patellar tendon, and an adjacent tibial ossicle (**Fig. 16**). Typically, tenderness is experienced both on palpation and with transducer pressure during ultrasound examination.

Patellar Bursitis

Three common bursae are related to the extensor mechanism: the prepatellar (housemaid's knee),

superficial, and deep infrapatellar bursae. In normal individuals, the prepatellar and superficial patellar bursae are not visualized on ultrasound, but occasionally a trace of fluid may be seen in the deep infrapatellar bursa. Inflammation and enlargement of the bursa relates to several predisposing causes, including trauma/hemorrhage, infection, gout, and rheumatoid arthritis.[4,5] On ultrasound examination, an enlarged bursa containing either simple or, more likely, complex fluid is visualized (**Figs. 17** and **18**). The bursa can normally be easily aspirated with ultrasound guidance on clinical request.

Medial Collateral Ligament Tear

Medial collateral ligament tear is usually associated with other injury to the knee, particularly anterior cruciate ligament injury and meniscal injury, and is normally examined with MR imaging. Isolated rupture of the MCL through pure valgus force is much less common. Acute injury to the MCL is

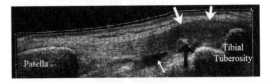

Fig. 16. Distal patellar tendonosis. Longitudinal image of the patellar tendon shows diffuse hypoechogenicity and some swelling of the distal tendon at and near the insertion on the tibial tuberosity (*short white wide arrows*). Note also the small amount of fluid in the deep infrapatellar bursa (*short thin white arrow*) and the small fragment of bone (*long black arrow*). The findings are consistent with Osgood-Schlatter changes. (*Courtesy of* J. Antonio Bouffard, MD, Detroit, MI.)

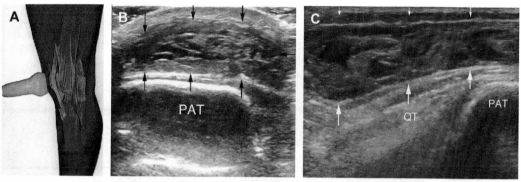

Fig. 17. Prepatellar bursitis. (A) Positioning of the transducer for the prepatellar bursa. (B, C) Transverse and longitudinal views show a distended prepatellar bursa containing complex fluid (*arrows*). Notice the bursa extends over the superior aspect of the patella and over the distal quadriceps tendon. QT, quadriceps tendon; PAT, patella.

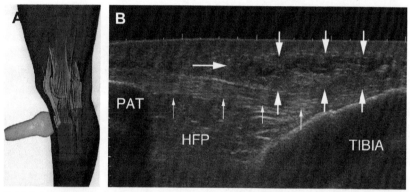

Fig. 18. Superficial infrapatellar bursitis. (A) Normal positioning of the transducer for the superficial and deep intrapatellar bursae. (B) Longitudinal image shows a distended superficial infrapatellar bursa (*large arrows*). Note the normal patellar tendon (*small arrows*). HFP, Hoffa's fat pad; PAT, patella; TIBIA, tibia.

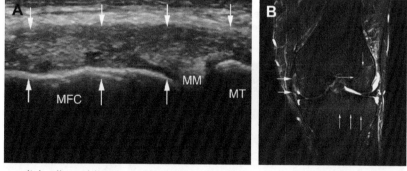

Fig. 19. Acute medial collateral ligament (MCL) tear. (A) Longitudinal image through the medial knee shows diffuse swelling of both the superficial and deep part of the MCL adjacent to the medial femoral condyle, consistent with an acute tear (*arrows*). Compare the appearances with the normal MCL in Fig. 10. MFC, medial femoral condyle; MM, medial meniscus; MT, medial tibia. (B) Coronal fat-suppressed T2-weighted image through the knee in the same patient shows the grade 2 tear of the MCL (*thick arrows*). Note also the bone edema laterally in the femoral and tibial condyles (*thin arrows*) consistent with valgus force. In this case, the MCL injury was consistent with pure valgus force, because no associated anterior cruciate ligament tear was present to suggest a rotatory component.

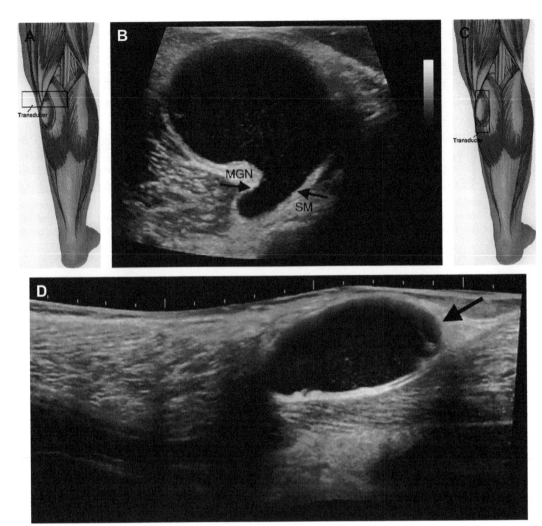

Fig. 20. Baker cyst. (*A*) Positioning of the transducer in the axial plane for imaging a Baker cyst. (*B*) Corresponding transverse ultrasound image shows the Baker cyst and, in particular, the neck of the cyst (*arrows*) between the medial head of the gastrocnemius and the semimembranosus. To diagnose a Baker cyst on ultrasound examination, the neck of the cyst must always be identified. MGN, medial head of the gastrocnemius; SM, semimembranosus. (*C*) Normal positioning for the longitudinal image. (*D*) Longitudinal image through the Baker cyst shows the cyst with a smooth inferior margin (*arrow*) between the medial gastrocnemius and the adjacent superficial fascia.

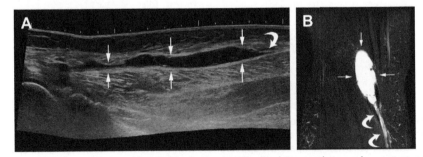

Fig. 21. Ruptured Baker cyst. (*A*) Extended field of view longitudinal image shows a large ruptured Baker cyst (*arrows*). Note the irregular margin of the inferior portion of the cyst (*curved arrow*) consistent with rupture. Contrast this appearance with that in **Fig. 20**D. The neck of the cyst was identified on axial imaging. (*B*) Corresponding MR image in the same patient. Coronal fast fat-suppressed T2-weighted image shows the Baker cyst (*straight arrows*) and the inferior rupture (*curved arrows*).

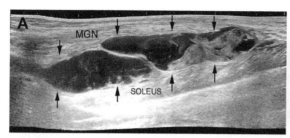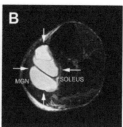

Fig. 22. Complex ruptured Baker cyst. (*A*) Longitudinal extended field of view image shows a complex mass in the calf between the medial gastrocnemius (MGN) muscle and the adjacent soleus (*arrows*). Findings suggested the neck of a Baker cyst on axial imaging. (*B*) Axial fat-saturated T2-weighted image through the calf shows a complex cystic collection between the MGN muscle and the adjacent soleus (*arrows*). The collection could be traced up to a neck between the medial head of the gastrocnemius muscle and the semimembranosus.

seen on ultrasound as loss of the normal fibrillar appearance of the ligament; swelling of the ligament, particularly the femoral origin; and discontinuity of the ligament (**Fig. 19**).

Baker Cyst and Ruptured Baker Cyst

Baker cyst is very common at the knee joint (**Fig. 20**). The slit-like neck of the cyst, between the medial head of the gastrocnemius and the semimembranosus, must be identified to establish the diagnosis, because other cyst-like masses around the knee, including tumors, may mimic a Baker cyst. Baker cysts are associated with increased intra-articular fluid and inflammatory arthropathies.[5] The cyst may contain simple or complex appearing fluid, synovium, and, in some cases, joint bodies.

Acute rupture of a Baker cyst is typically painful, with the patient experiencing calf pain and swelling. Occasionally, acute rupture of a Baker cyst may be very disabling, with the patient's mobility hindered by the severe pain and discomfort. Ruptured Baker cysts can present clinically with symptoms similar to a deep vein thrombosis. On ultrasound examination, rupture is characterized by irregularity of the inferior margin of the cyst (**Fig. 21**). Occasionally, the cyst can dissect between the medial gastrocnemius and the soleus (**Fig. 22**).

Knee Joint Effusion

Ultrasound is very sensitive in detecting knee joint effusions. Usually minimal to no fluid is seen within the suprapatellar bursa on ultrasound examination. Fluid is seen in varying amounts accumulating between the prefemoral fat, suprapatellar fat pad, and the quadriceps tendon (**Fig. 23**). Fluid may be simple-appearing or

anechoic, or complex with echoes within it. In the setting of possible septic arthritis, whether fluid is infected cannot be determined using ultrasound criteria; aspiration with laboratory analysis is required.

Ultrasound is ideally suited to aspirate a knee joint effusion (**Fig. 24**). First, whether a knee joint effusion is present can be determined with ultrasound. Second, the aspiration can be performed under ultrasound guidance. The suprapatellar bursa is tapped in the setting of knee joint effusion with the clinical request for aspiration. The authors use sterile technique, including covering the transducer with a sterile cover, and perform the procedure in "real time," with the needle being followed into the joint. The bursa usually can be tapped at the medial or lateral margin of the suprapatellar bursa (see **Fig. 24**).

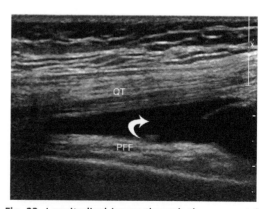

Fig. 23. Longitudinal image through the suprapatellar bursa shows a large joint effusion (*curved arrow*); contrast this appearance with that in **Fig. 1**. QT, quadriceps tendon; PFF, prefemoral fat.

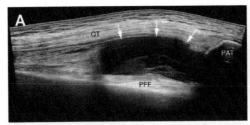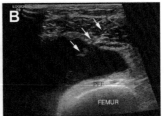

Fig. 24. (*A*) Longitudinal image through the knee shows a markedly distended suprapatellar bursa (*arrows*). QT, quadriceps tendon; PAT, patellar; PFF, prefemoral fat. (*B*) Aspiration of the knee from a medial approach, medial to the quadriceps tendon. Note the needle (*arrows*). PFF, prefemoral fat.

SUMMARY

Advanced imaging of the knee joint is most commonly performed using MR imaging. Ultrasound can display much of the normal knee anatomy but has major limitations in assessment of the meniscus and cruciate ligaments and cannot image through cortex/subchondral bone. However, in evaluating knee joint effusion and ultrasound-guided aspiration, ultrasound is unsurpassed. In the clinical setting of rupture of the quadriceps tendon or patellar tendon, it is very useful, as it is in assessment and rupture of Baker cyst.

ACKNOWLEDGMENTS

The authors thank Jay Knipstein for the illustrations.

REFERENCES

1. Gardner E, Gray DS, O'Rahilly R. Thigh and knee. In: Anatomy. 4th edition. Philadelphia: WB Saunders; 1975. p. 210–26.
2. van Holsbeeck MT, Introcasso JH. Sonography of ligaments. In: Musculoskeletal ultrasound. 2nd edition. St. Louis (MO): Mosby; 2001. p. 171–92.
3. Rogers LF. The knee and shafts of the tibia and fibula. In: Radiology of skeletal trauma. 2nd edition. New York: Churchill Livingstone; 1992. p. 1269–70.
4. Resnick D, Kang HS. Knee. In: Internal derangement of joints. Philadelphia: WB Saunders; 1997. p. 555–785.
5. van Holsbeeck MT, Introcasso JH. Sonography of bursae. In: Musculoskeletal ultrasound. 2nd edition. St. Louis (MO): Mosby; 2001. p. 131–69.

Ultrasound of the Foot and Ankle

Kil-Ho Cho, MD, PhDa,*,
Gervais Khin-Lin Wansaicheong, MBBS, FRCR, MMed (Diagnostic Radiology)b

KEYWORDS

- Musculoskeletal • Ultrasound • Ankle • Foot • Anatomy • Pathology

KEY POINTS

- Accurate diagnosis of pathology in the ankle and foot depends on understanding the anatomy.
- Dynamic evaluation is helpful, as it can reveal abnormalities that are inadequate on static imaging and can correlate symptoms with the site of sonographic findings.
- With ultrasound, tendon and ligament diseases are easily diagnosed and distinguished from other peri-articular and intra-articular diseases.
- Ultrasound can be used as a potential tool for determining further radiological evaluation and for image-guiding interventional procedures.

Symptomatic ankle and foot ailments are usually diagnosed on the basis of medical history, physical examination, and radiography. Currently, ultrasound (US) is used as the second-line imaging modality after radiography because it can depict soft tissue structures that are not well visualized on radiography.[1] A unique advantage of US is real-time dynamic evaluation, which can reveal abnormalities that are inadequately delineated on static imaging. With US, it is easy to compare the symptomatic area to the asymptomatic opposite side. Additional information can be obtained during the scanning while interacting with the patient.[2] To perform and understand US findings of various injuries and pathology in the ankle and foot,[3] it is essential to know detailed US anatomy, artifacts, exact probe positioning, and limitations.

ANATOMY AND PATHOLOGY OF THE ANKLE

The anatomic structures of the ankle can be divided into 4 groups (anterior, medial, lateral, and posterior) (**Fig. 1**).[4] Pathology that is commonly seen in each group is described after the anatomy in the following sections.

Posterior Aspect

The Achilles (or calcaneal) tendon is the largest and strongest tendon in the body. It is capable of withstanding forces 12 times the body weight during running or jumping.[5] The tendon usually measures 10 to 15 cm long with a uniform thickness of 4 to 7 mm.[6] The tendon does not have a tendon sheath, but is surrounded by a paratenon. The Achilles tendon is composed of 3 twisted different fascicles coming from the triceps surae muscle (the medial and lateral heads of the gastrocnemius, soleus, and plantaris). The posterior lateral one-third of the tendon is composed of collagenous fibers from the medial head of the gastrocnemius muscle, the anterior lateral third is composed of fibers from the lateral head of the gastrocnemius, and the central third and medial part are composed of fibers from the soleus muscle (**Fig. 2**).[7] Rupture

Funding sources: Nil. Conflict of interest: Nil.
a Department of Diagnostic Radiology, Yeungnam University Hospital, School of Medicine, Yeungnam University, 317-1, Daemyung-Dong, Nam-Gu, Daegu 705-717, Korea; b Department of Diagnostic Radiology, Tan Tock Seng Hospital, 11 Jalan Tan Tock Seng, Singapore 308433, Singapore
* Corresponding author.
E-mail address: Khcho.med@ynu.ac.kr

ultrasound.theclinics.com

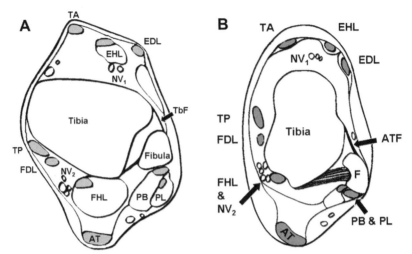

Fig. 1. (*A*) Line diagram of a cross section of the left ankle at the level of the inferior tibiofibular ligaments shows the ankle tendons. The Achilles tendon (AT) is situated posteriorly. The anterior neurovascular bundle (NV₁) consists of the anterior tibial artery and deep peroneal nerve. The medial neurovascular bundle (NV₂) consists of the posterior tibial artery and tibial nerve. The other tendons and labels have been labeled with the same abbreviations used in the text. (*B*) Line diagram of a cross section of the left ankle at the level of the anterior talofibular ligaments shows the ankle tendons. This is inferior to the section in **Fig. 1A**. The peroneus brevis tendon lies against the fibula and is larger than the peroneus longus. The fibula is labeled as F. *Abbreviation:* ATF, Anterior Talo-Fibular ligament; EDL, Extensor Digitorum Longus tendon; EHL, Extensor Hallucis Longus tendon; FDL, Flexor Digitorum Longus tendon; FHL, Felxor Hallucis Longus tendon; PB, Peroneus Brevis tendon; PL, Peroneus Longus tendon; TA, Tibialis Anterior tendon; TbF, anterior Tibio-Fibular ligament; TP, Tibialis Posterior tendon.

most commonly occurs in the distal 2 to 6 cm of the tendon (watershed zone). The slender plantaris tendon (absent in up to 20% of individuals) courses just medial to the Achilles tendon. Both the Achilles and plantaris tendons insert onto the posterior calcaneal tuberosity.[8]

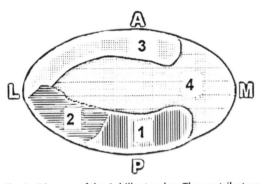

Fig. 2. Diagram of the Achilles tendon. The contributors of the tendon twist are (1) the fibers from the medial part of the medial head of the gastrocnemius, (2) the fibers from the lateral part of the medial head of the gastrocnemius, (3) the fibers from the lateral head of the gastrocnemius and (4) the fibers from the soleus. The orientation of the tendon is marked A: anterior, P: posterior, M: medial, L: lateral. (*Adapted from* Szaro P, Witkowski G, Smigielski R, et al. Fascicles of the adult human Achilles tendon-anatomic study. Annals Ana 2009;191:590; with permission.)

The Achilles tendon in long-axis view shows a typical hyperechoic fibrillar pattern that is similar to any other tendon in the body. If the insonating sound beam is not perpendicular to the tendon, the fibers may appear hypoechoic or even anechoic because of the anisotropy artifact. This artifact should be avoided as much as possible by changing the angle of the transducer to maintain a perpendicular orientation of the sound beam to the tendon. The insertion of the Achilles tendon in longitudinal view is usually hypoechoic owing to anisotropy (**Fig. 3**).

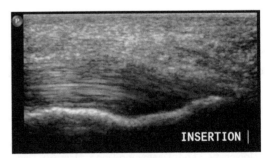

Fig. 3. US image of the Achilles tendon. The tendon inserts onto the posterior aspect of the calcaneus. Anisotropy is noted at the distal end of the tendon as the tendon fibers curve and insert onto the posterior calcaneal tuberosity.

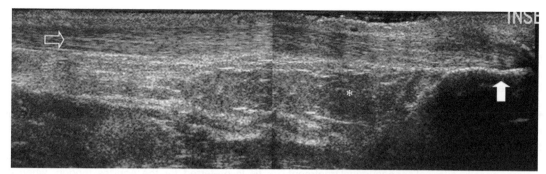

Fig. 4. US image of the Achilles tendon (*empty arrow*). Kager's fat pad is seen deep to the tendon (*white asterisk*). The posterior calcaneal tuberosity is indicated with the *white arrow*.

A triangular hyperechoic fat-filled space known as the Kager fat pad (**Fig. 4**) is found anterior to the Achilles tendon and posterior to the distal tibia and flexor hallucis longus.[8] The retrocalcaneal (or pre-Achilles) bursa is a thin anechoic slit (containing fluid with an anteroposterior distance up to 2.5 mm) between the distal Achilles tendon and the posterior calcaneal tuberosity. Posterior to the Achilles tendon lies the subcutaneous bursa.

The accessory soleus muscle, a normal variant, can cause fullness with distortion of the Kager fat pad in the posteromedial aspect of the ankle.[9] This can mimic a tumorous condition. Another normal variant is the os trigonum, an accessory ossicle, which is found posterior to the posterior talocalcaneal joint. These variants should not be regarded as pathology.

Acute rupture of Achilles tendon commonly occurs in middle-aged men and about 60% of cases are related to a sports injury.[10] More than 20% of full-thickness tears can be missed clinically at initial presentation. Edema, hematoma, and pain in an acute tear can obliterate a tendon defect, which renders palpation ineffective.[11] Thus, there is a need for a rapid and reliable means of diagnosing full-thickness tears. The examiner can usually palpate a gap at the site of the tear, and can demonstrate decreased plantar flexion actively or passively with a calf squeeze (Thompson test). US findings of a complete tear include an anechoic fluid or a blood-filled defect at the site of the tear with retraction and swelling of the torn ends (**Fig. 5**). The Kager fat pad may herniate into the defect at the torn site of the tendon. In a partial

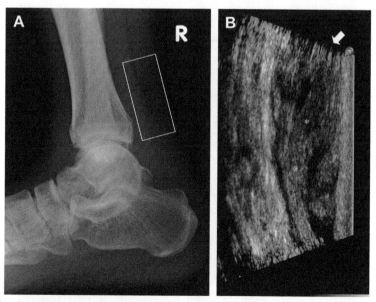

Fig. 5. (*A*) Lateral radiograph of the ankle shows a discontinuity in the outline of the Achilles tendon within the empty white box. (*B*) Corresponding US image of the Achilles tendon. The image has been rotated 90° to the right to match the white box in the radiograph of **Fig. 4A**. The normal tendon fibers (*white arrow*) show disruption of the normal fibrillar pattern (*white asterisk*).

tear, only a part of the tendon is frayed. There is hypoechoic discontinuity of the normal hyperechoic fibrillar pattern and the tendon is slightly thickened. Dynamic evaluation with passive motion is helpful in differentiation of a partial tear from a complete tear. The Thompson test is also useful in differentiating a plantaris tendon rupture from an Achilles tendon rupture. The test is negative (ie, there is normal plantar flexion) in the case of a plantaris tendon tear. Distinguishing between these 2 conditions is important because an Achilles rupture requires specific surgical or nonsurgical treatment, but a plantaris tendon rupture requires only symptomatic treatment.

Achilles tendinopathy presents as local pain and tenderness exacerbated by activity. The pain is often in the heel or just proximal to it.[12] It is common in runners (up to 11%).[13] A variety of terms (tendinitis, tendinosis, tendinopathy, tendon degeneration, paratendinitis, and tenosynovitis)

have been used to describe tendon-related abnormalities. Although the term tendinitis is a common description to various medical professionals, there is no inflammation histopathologically. Thus, the term tendinopathy is recommended for the clinical diagnosis describing overuse tendon conditions with pain, swelling, and decreased function.[14,15] The term tendinosis means degeneration or structural change on histopathology. In fact, inflammation is often predominant in the peritendinous tissues instead. In this situation, paratendinitis is preferred for the Achilles tendon, whereas tenosynovitis for any tendon when tendon sheath is present.

A difference in the anteroposterior dimension of 2 mm or more between the right and left Achilles tendons is considered significant and is suggestive of tendinopathy. In chronic tendinopathy, calcification is rarely found. Tendon thickening (more than 8 mm) and circumscribed hypoechoic alteration of

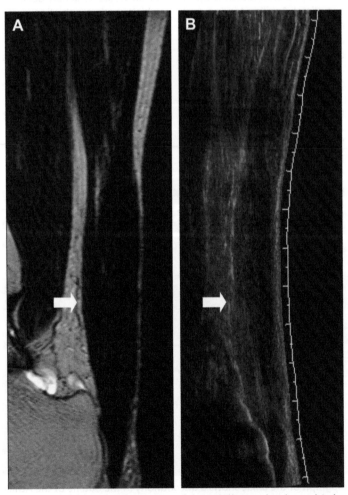

Fig. 6. (A) Sagittal T2-weighted MR image of thickening of the Achilles tendon (arrow) in hypercholesterolaemia. (B) The corresponding US image has been rotated to match the diffusely thickened hypoechoic area (arrow) of the tendon with the hypointense tendon.

echotexture on US are associated with a significantly higher rate of tendon rupture and worse clinical outcome on follow-up.[16] In patients with familial hypercholesterolemia, US can detect Achilles tendon xanthomas (**Fig. 6**). The imaging finding can range from single hypoechoic nodules to diffusely enlarged, heterogeneously hypoechoic tendons. These findings may simulate partial tendon tears or tendinosis.

Retrocalcaneal bursitis presents with similar symptoms.[17] Retrocalcaneal (= sub-Achilles) bursitis arises most commonly from overuse injury but also may develop in systemic diseases, such as rheumatoid or seronegative spondyloarthropathies (**Fig. 7**). Superficial Achilles (= subcutaneous) bursa may be inflamed owing to local irritation, for example, from the upper edge of a rigid shoe counter (**Fig. 8**). Lateral malleolar bursitis is more common, and may become enlarged in gout.[18] Chronic perimalleolar pain is not always caused by tendon tear. Scar formation in the tendons, capsules, and ligaments; tenosynovitis or chronic bursitis around the ankle; or tumors can also cause swelling and pain. Nodular or fusiform swelling of the tendon may suggest a partial tear combined with tendinopathy. Microscopically, alteration of tenocytes and collagen fibers by longitudinal splitting and mucoid degeneration with disintegrated tendon structures has been found in 97% of patients with spontaneously ruptured tendons.[19] It is often overlooked initially because the patient has relatively little pain and walks after the rupture. Insertional Achilles tendinopathy may develop from microtears that give rise to chronic inflammation, a mucinous degenerating nodule, calcium deposits, and even complete tears (**Fig. 9**A). The Haglund deformity is a painful posterior bump at

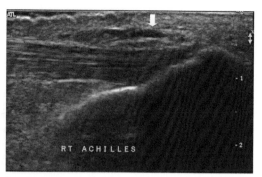

Fig. 8. US image of the superficial Achilles bursa distended with fluid (*white arrow*).

the level of the superior calcaneal margin, caused by excessive compression of the Achilles tendon. A symptom complex with all 3 entities mentioned previously is called Haglund syndrome.[20] US can reveal localized thickening of the skin and subcutaneous tissue, peritendinous bursal distention, and calcified insertion enthesopathy (see **Fig. 9**B). US may be able to make the distinction between tendinopathy and bursitis, and is very helpful for injection of steroid for the treatment of bursitis and avoiding an inappropriate injection of steroid into the tendon itself.

The term "overuse syndrome" refers to an injury resulting from an excessive repetition of a common activity or an injury as a result of performance of an activity to which an individual is not accustomed.[12] Most overuse syndromes are the result of repetitive minor insults. The ability of individuals to tolerate and repair these insults varies considerably. The etiologies of these insults include mechanical trauma and nontraumatic causes like anatomic variants and metabolic and vascular diseases. The syndrome is commonly associated with sporting activities, such as cycling, ice skating, ballet, and running. Acute severe trauma causes musculotendinous junction disruption or fracture. Although nearly all tendinous injuries can be evaluated with US, not all the patients with acute ankle injuries need to be evaluated with US. It may be used in patients suspected of having a tendon rupture or inflammation or in patients with persistent pain and swelling lasting longer than 4 weeks.

Anterior Aspect

Anteriorly, the 3 tendons related to dorsiflexion of the ankle run superiorly to inferiorly in individual compartments. The tibialis anterior (TA) tendon is located medially and lies anterior to the medial malleolus, next to the great saphenous vein. The TA tendon provides 80% of the dorsiflexion power of the ankle, and is the second strongest tendon after the Achilles tendon (**Fig. 10**A). Moving

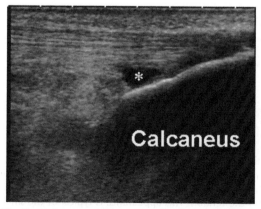

Fig. 7. US image of the pre-Achilles bursa distended with fluid (*). Small amounts of fluid are considered physiologic. However, larger amounts that are associated with increased vascularity or pain on compression are considered typical of bursitis.

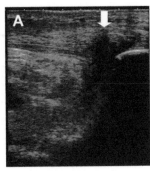
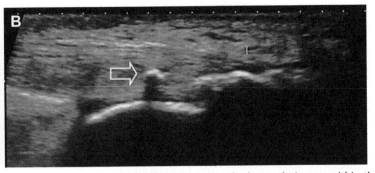

Fig. 9. (A) US image of the Achilles tendon with insertional tendinopathy. Note the hypoechoic area within the tendon substance and thickening of the tendon (*white arrow*). (B) US image of the Achilles tendon with calcific enthesopathy (*empty arrow*).

laterally, the next 2 tendons are the extensor hallucis longus (EHL) and the extensor digitorum longus (EDL). The anterior tibial artery and deep peroneal nerve lie between the EHL and EDL tendons (see **Fig. 10B**). Fluid is rarely seen around the anterior tendons (2% of population). In particular, fluid in the distal 1 to 2 cm of the TA tendon is almost always regarded as pathologic. Physiologic fluid in the joint is common in asymptomatic patients, and the amount of fluid is not significantly different in patients with symptoms. The examiners, therefore, should be careful before diagnosing diseases based on the presence of fluid in the ankle.[21,22]

The anterior tendons of the ankle are rarely injured.[23] The anterior tibial tendon has a straight course and minimal mechanical demands. This is consistent with its rare involvement by inflammation or rupture. In patients with a previous fracture, degenerative arthritis, or other predisposing factors, tendon rupture can occur. Chronic inflammation or more significant involvement is seen in runners. The toe extensors (EHL and EDL) generate little force and there is minimal physical

disability associated with rupture. Local pressure on the dorsum of the foot and ankle from tight footwear or shoelaces may cause pain caused by extensor synovitis, anterior tibial neuritis, or a combination of both. US may be helpful in differentiating tendon edema or tendon sheath swelling from tendon rupture.

Lateral Aspect

Two tendons (peroneus brevis and longus) are located in the posterior fibular (or retro-malleolar) groove of the lateral malleolus. They pronate and evert the foot, and help perform the second stage of walking and push-off. They share a common tendon sheath at the malleolar level. This appears as a "figure 8" or snowman on US. Normal tendons may be surrounded by a halo of fluid no more than 2 mm thick. The peroneus brevis (PB) tendon is seen as pancake shaped and close to the lateral malleolus, whereas the peroneus longus (PL) tendon is ovoid and superficial to the PB tendon. This normal relationship is lost if there

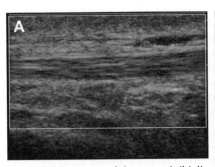
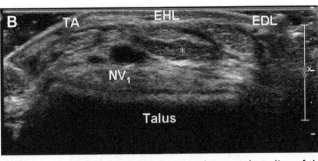

Fig. 10. (A) US image of the normal tibialis anterior tendon in longitudinal axis. Note the smooth outline of the tendon sheath seen as a continuous hyperechoic line. The tendon itself consists of parallel short to medium length echogenic lines. No vascularity is noted in or around the tendon. This appearance is typical of the small tendons around the ankle. (B) US image of the tibialis anterior tendon in transverse (or short) axis at the level of the talus, just distal to the level shown in **Fig. 1B**. Note that just deep to the tendon of the EHL, part of the muscle belly (*white asterisk*) is still seen. As the different tendons are similar in longitudinal axis, it is useful to check the position of the tendon in the short axis to confirm its identity. The tendons have been labeled with the same abbreviations used in the text.

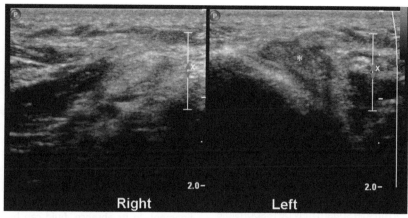

Fig. 11. US image of the peroneal tendons in transverse (or short) axis with altered echogenicity in the peroneus brevis tendon (*white asterisk*). A side-by-side comparison has been obtained to demonstrate the tendinosis of the left side.

is subluxation of the tendon. Subluxation that is not apparent at rest can be elicited by dynamic stress maneuver (combined dorsiflexion and eversion) of the foot.[24] The PB and PL tendons diverge at the infra-malleolar level with each tendon having a separate tendon sheath. Normally a small amount of fluid is seen in the tendon sheath (in 16%–17% of population).[21]

The PB tendon inserts onto the base of the fifth metatarsal head; and the PL tendon, onto the base of the first metatarsal and the medial cuneiform. As a normal variant, an accessory tendon called the peroneus quartus, may be found posterior to the fibula; this tendon most commonly originates from the PB and inserts on the lateral aspect of the calcaneus at the retrotrochlear eminence.

The peroneal tendons, theoretically, should be susceptible to tendinitis and rupture within the pulley where they undergo an acute change in direction. However, pathology is rare (**Fig. 11**). Peroneal injury is one of the major complications of intra-articular calcaneal fracture. Longitudinal tears (also called "peroneal splits") are more common in the PB tendon because of increased stress on this tendon as it is trapped between the PL tendon and the fibula. Subluxation or dislocation of the peroneal tendons is seen acutely when there is rupture of the peroneal retinaculum in dorsiflexion/eversion injuries or calcaneal fractures.

The ligamentous structures in the lateral aspect of the ankle consist of the anterior inferior tibiofibular (TbF) ligament, and the lateral collateral ligament (LCL) complex (**Fig. 12**). The TbF ligament between the distal tibia and fibula is 2 to 3 mm thick, 11 to 20 mm long, and 6 to 10 mm wide in the middle part.[25] The TbF ligament's most important function is to prevent anterior diastasis between the 2 bones. Anterior diastasis may be

caused by an external rotation force at the ankle, resulting in an exaggerated external rotation and posterior translation of the fibula with respect to tibia following loss of the anterior inferior TbF ligament. Surgical treatment is necessary for most conditions because of instability.[26]

The 3 components of the LCL complex are the anterior talofibular (ATF), posterior talofibular (PTF), and calcaneofibular (CF) ligaments. On US, the ankle ligaments are 2 to 3 mm thick by the authors' experience. Anatomically, the ATF ligament (9–12 mm wide; and 20–25 mm long in the middle part)[27] runs from the anterior inferior aspect of the fibula to the lateral anterior surface

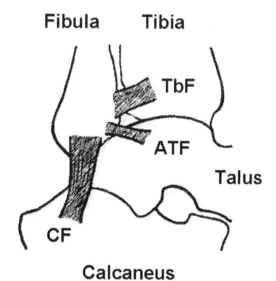

Fig. 12. Line diagram of the lateral view of the ankle shows the ligaments that are sonographically visible. The ligaments have been labeled with the same abbreviations used in the text.

of the talus (**Fig. 13**). It is considered the most vulnerable among the ankle ligaments. The CF ligament (28–35 mm long, and 3–6 mm wide in the middle part)[27] takes an oblique course from the tip of the fibula caudally and slightly posterior to the lateral aspect of the calcaneus. It passes deep to the 2 peroneus tendons. The PTF, posterior inferior TbF, and the transverse ligaments are too deep to be depicted with US.

Ligament Injury

The only abnormality on standard radiographs for ligamentous injuries may be soft tissue swelling. The presence of muscle spasm may be responsible for a falsely normal test. If arthrography, an invasive method, is performed for diagnosis, it should be done as soon as possible after injury. False-negative results may occur owing to sealing of the capsular defect. US may detect an intraligamentous partial tear that is undetectable with arthroscopy because the latter can evaluate only the visible surface of the ligament.[28] Most foot and ankle ligamentous injuries are related to sporting, gymnastics, and aerobic activities. Imaging of ligament injuries of the foot and ankle is difficult. Ultrasonically painful nodular granulation tissue can be detected at the site of ligamentous lesions after inadequate or absent treatment.

The most frequent injury referred for US in the ankle is the lateral ankle sprain. Clinically, this presents with a variable degree of pain, swelling, and ecchymosis. The mechanism of the injury is considerably controversial. The typical ankle sprain is caused by internal rotation, plantar flexion, and adduction of the talus beyond its physiologic limit. The ATF ligament and adjacent joint capsule are usually ruptured (**Fig. 14**)[29]; with persistent force, the secondary restraints (CF

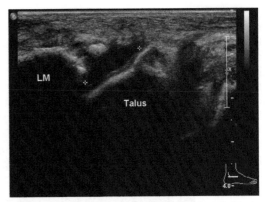

Fig. 14. US image of a complete tear of the talofibular ligament. In its absence, fluid can be seen between the calipers and below the LM.

and PTF ligaments) are also injured. This results in severe talar instability.

In 70% of lateral ankle sprains, only the ATF ligament is torn; the CF ligament is also torn in 20% of the cases. The resultant injury is commonly accompanied with an avulsion fracture of the distal fibula (**Fig. 15**). A tear of the anterior TbF ligament is difficult to detect on physical examination and radiography alone. There may be no talar tilt on

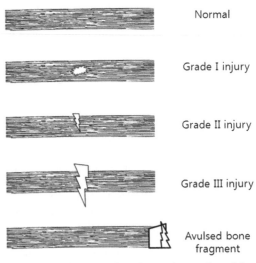

Fig. 15. Line diagram that shows the grades of ligament injury of the lateral collateral ligaments. Grade I: Stretch with partial ligamentous fibrillar fault or tear without disruption or instability. It presents with mild swelling, pain, and tenderness over the ATF ligament. Grade II: An incomplete ligamentous disruption with overall continuity maintained. The utility of physical examination is limited to in this setting. Discomfort over the CF ligament is not uncommon. Grade III: Full-thickness tear of the ligament has occurred, resulting in ankle instability. An avulsed bone fragments may be seen in more severe cases.

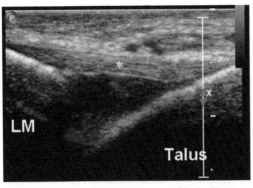

Fig. 13. US image of the anterior talofibular ligament (*white asterisk*). It can be seen running from the lateral malleolus (LM) to the talus.

routine radiographs. The PTF ligament is almost never torn, as an avulsion fracture occurs before ligamentous rupture. For the treatment of ankle sprain, rest and support to the area (3–8 weeks) is usually required until pain, soreness, and tenderness are no longer elicited.[30] When chronic discomfort and swelling are present for more than 6 weeks in patients diagnosed initially with an "ankle sprain," it is important to consider the possibility of other significant pathology and to perform a magnetic resonance (MR) scan as the next step in imaging.[31]

Medial Aspect

Medially, the tibialis posterior (TP), the flexor digitorum longus (FDL), and the flexor hallucis longus (FHL) tendons are found from an anterior to posterior position (see **Fig. 1**A). At the malleolar level, the cross-sectional area of the TP is roughly twice that of the FDL. The TP tendon has a complex insertion onto the navicular, 3 cuneiforms, and bases of the second to fourth metatarsal bones. The FDL follows a path just posterior and lateral to the TP and inserts on the plantar aspects of the bases of distal phalanges 2 through 5. A neurovascular bundle (posterior tibial artery and vein, and tibial nerve) is located between the FDL and FHL tendon.

The flexor retinaculum extends from the medial malleolus to the calcaneus, superficial to the foregoing structures, to form the roof of the tarsal tunnel. The anatomy of the structures within the tarsal tunnel (from anterior to posterior) is easily remembered with the mnemonic "Tom, Dick, And Very Nervous Harry," which stands for Tibialis tendon, Digitorum tendon, Artery, Veins, Nerve, and Hallucis tendon. The tibial nerve divides into medial and lateral plantar branches. These continue toward the digits as the common plantar digital nerves and then as the proper plantar digital nerves.

Passing deeply posterior to the distal tibia, the FHL tendon enters a shallow groove in the medial posterior aspect of the talus. Then the tendon takes a curved course under the plantar surface of the sustentaculum tali of the calcaneus, passes between sesamoids at the base of the first metatarsal head, and inserts onto the great toe. The FHL has been called the "Achilles tendon" of ballet dancers. In the plantar aspect in the midfoot, the FDL and FHL tendons cross each other, a configuration termed the knot of Henry. Fluid in tendon sheaths around the ankle is normally seen along the TP (22% of population), the FDL (24%), and the FHL (31%) tendons.[22] Although tendon fluid may be present in asymptomatic ankles, fluid in the distal 1 to 2 cm of the tendon is always abnormal (**Fig. 16**).

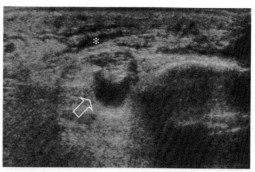

Fig. 16. US image of the medial tendons of the ankle. Note the fluid around the posterior tibial tendon (*empty arrow*). Subcutaneous edema is seen (*white asterisk*).

The medial collateral ligament (MCL) of the ankle has many synonyms. It is more commonly known as the deltoid ligament. It lies beneath the TP and FDL tendons and consists of 3 superficial (tibionavicular, tibiocalcaneal, and superficial tibiotalar) and 2 deep (anterior tibiotalar and posterior tibiotalar) components. The deltoid ligaments are infrequently injured compared with the lateral ankle ligaments.

Usually, US is focused on the symptomatic area that is relevant to the patient's history or as directed by the patient. This is often a clue in localizing lesions that are not routinely assessed. A complete examination of all areas should be considered if no pathology is found because there are many closely associated structures that may produce similar symptoms.

The TP tendon is the most commonly injured among the medial ankle tendons. Shear load can cause transverse rupture of the tendon at the point between the medial malleolus and navicular bone. Such a tear leads to progressive flatfoot deformity and weakness on inversion of the foot. When the TP tendon is torn, the action of the antagonist muscle (PB tendon) is unopposed, resulting in a planovalgar deformity of the foot. US can assess tendon integrity directly, and secondary signs, including tenosynovitis and surrounding edema (**Fig. 17**).[32] Acute traumatic rupture of the posterior tibial tendon is associated with medial malleolar fractures. The tendon may be torn longitudinally; this presents with elongated swelling and intratendinous hypoechoic cleavages on US. Rupture of the FDL and FHL tendons occurs less frequently than the TP tendon but can present with similar clinical findings.

Tendon disorders of FHL or FDL may cause pain in the posteromedial aspect of the ankle or along the plantar aspect of the midfoot. Toe flexors tendinopathy or tendon rupture may be a significant clinical problem, for example in a classic ballet

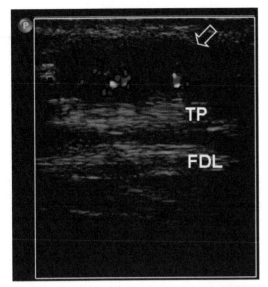

Fig. 17. US image of thickened synovium (*open arrow*) around the tibialis (TP) tendon. Note the increased flow on color Doppler imaging and the deep position of the flexor digitorum longus (FDL) tendon.

dancer in whom a high force is generated within the FHL to accomplish and maintain a toe raise.[33]

Inferior Aspect

The plantar fascia attaches to the anterior aspect of the inferior surface of the calcaneus, which normally measures 3 to 4 mm thick at the calcaneal attachment (**Fig. 18A**). Like tendons, the plantar fascia can also exhibit anisotropic artifact.

Plantar fasciitis, representing inflammation of the fascia and its surrounding structures caused by stress of repetitive trauma, is one of the most common causes of heel pain. A pathognomonic feature is pain and tenderness at the medial tubercle of the calcaneus where the central and thickest portion of the plantar fascia is attached. The plantar fascia becomes hypoechoic, and shows fusiform thickening (5–10 mm), compared with asymptomatic patients in whom the fascia is hyperechoic and flat (see **Fig. 18B**).[34] Occasionally patients with symptoms that are refractory to conservative management are considered for surgery (fasciotomy at the calcaneal attachment). Arthropathies that predispose to plantar fasciitis include seronegative variants of rheumatoid arthritis.

Plantar fibromatosis (or Ledderhose disease) affects 1% to 2% of the general population. Most occur in the fourth decade. The etiology is unknown and the age of onset is variable. There is benign fibrous proliferation of the plantar fascia. On US, the plantar fascia nodularity is hypoechoic and does not have a consistent relationship with the calcaneal attachment of the fascia (**Fig. 19**).[35] The best method of evaluating these patients is MR imaging (MRI) with gadolinium enhancement.

PATHOLOGY COMMON TO THE ANKLE AND FOOT
Articular Cartilage and Ankle Joint

The tibiotalar (talocrural or ankle) joint is usually scanned from an anterior sagittal plane of the joint with the foot in plantar flexion. The dorsiflexor tendons of the ankle are located just under the

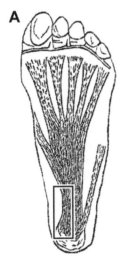

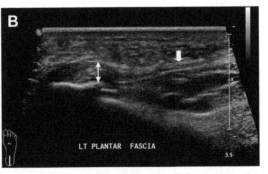

Fig. 18. (A) Line diagram of the plantar fascia. The thickening in plantar fasciitis is found in the area outlined by the box. (B) US image of a thickened plantar fascia. The measurement is made at the thickest portion of the fascia near the tip of the calcaneal bone (*double-headed white arrow*). The rest of the plantar fascia (*white arrow*) is normal in thickness.

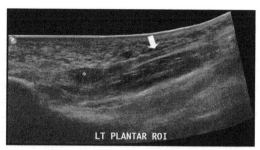

Fig. 19. US image of plantar fibromatosis. The nodule is marked with a *white asterisk*. The rest of the plantar fascia (*white arrow*) is normal in thickness. Note that the nodule lies away from the usual site of plantar fasciitis.

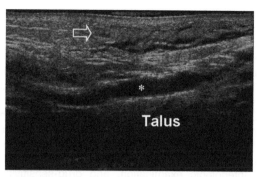

Fig. 21. US image of the anterior recess in a parasagittal plane. Note the anterior recess effusion (*white asterisk*). Subcutaneous edema (*empty arrow*) is present.

skin and the anterior joint is defined by the hyperechoic bone surface of the tibia and talus, and their hypoechoic articular hyaline cartilage, which is 1 to 2 mm thick. The space between the superficially located extensor tendons and bones is filled with triangular hyperechoic fat (so-called "normal delta sign") (**Fig. 20**). Normally, joint fluid less than 2 mm thick in anterior-posterior (AP) diameter is seen between the bone and fat. Physiologic fluid is found in the anterior recess of the ankle joint (60%), in the posterior recess of the ankle joint (77%), in the subtalar joint (72%), and less commonly in the anterior recess of the anterior talocalcaneal joint (29% of the population).[22] The hypoechoic articular cartilage and physiologic joint fluid should not be mistaken as pathologic effusion.

It is important to evaluate not only the anterior joint recess in the sagittal plane, but also the parasagittal plane, to look for small amounts of joint fluid (**Fig. 21**). Graded compression on the joint recesses with the free hand aids visualization of

intra-articular debris and fluid. This helps in the detection of small amounts of joint fluid, as solid tissue is usually not compressible.

In clinical practice, US can distinguish articular diseases from peri-articular conditions. There are 3 broad classes of joint pathology: (1) traumatic,

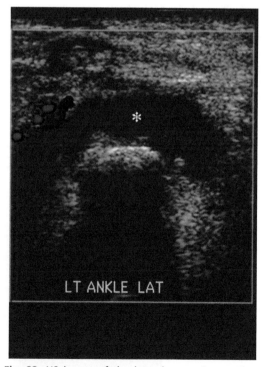

Fig. 22. US image of the lateral recess in a patient with septic arthritis of the ankle. There is increased vascularity in the surrounding tissue, subcutaneous edema, and thickening of the synovium and an effusion (*white asterisk*) in the lateral recess. Although the combination of features is suggestive of an infection, confirmation with an aspiration of the fluid can be extremely useful in obtaining a culture for diagnosis and sensitivity to antibiotics for treatment.

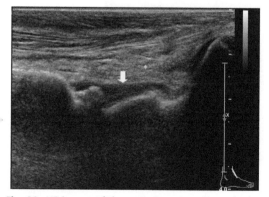

Fig. 20. US image of the anterior recess. Note the hyperechoic fat (*white asterisk*) and anterior recess (*white arrow*). An ankle effusion will expand the anterior recess and be compressible.

(2) inflammatory, and (3) infectious. Simple effusion is almost always anechoic; however, a variety of conditions, such as hemarthrosis, osteoarthrosis, inflammatory arthritides, and pyogenic or tuberculous arthritis, may have similar US findings: increased joint fluid with various echogenicity and synovial hyperplasia.[36–38] In this ambiguous clinical setting, percutaneous needle aspiration with or without biopsy of the joint lesions is essential for final diagnosis.[38] By the authors' experience, performing both the fluid aspiration (for cell count, bacteriologic examination, and drug-sensitivity) and biopsy (for histologic diagnosis) at one stage is more helpful, informative, and saves time (Fig. 22).

In patients with clinically symptomatic anterolateral ankle impingement, US can show synovitic lesions in excess of 10 mm within the anterolateral gutter of the ankle joint.[39] US can be extremely useful in detecting intra-articular loose bodies. These are usually associated with an effusion, regardless of the cause (traumatic or synovial chondromatosis, osteoarthritis, or crystalline arthritis). US can depict loose bodies as a hyperechoic crescent with posterior sonic shadowing, which are not visualized on radiography because of poor mineralization. A dynamic examination in the symptomatic area in active and passive joint motion can help to determine if a calcification is intra-articular.[40] In doubtful cases, US-guided intra-articular injection of small amount of sterile saline (less than 5–10 mL) may help in detecting tiny loose bodies, although it is invasive procedure.[41]

Bone abnormalities found during assessment of soft tissues or joints should be incorporated in the reporting of the US examination. Not only articular but peri-articular soft tissue diseases may cause bone changes. Erosion of cortical bone on US examination is seen as loss of the normal bright, linear hyperechoic surface.[36] Incidentally, thinning of the bone cortex with mirror-image artifact within the bone can be visualized in case of intra-osseous lesions, such as simple bone cyst (Fig. 23) or intra-osseous lipoma of the calcaneus.

The tophus in gout is seen as a hypoechoic nodule (± mild posterior shadowing), most commonly over the medial aspect of the first metatarsal head. Bone erosions may also be seen.[42] Extensor tendons can be surrounded by tophi. The tophi are hypoechoic because they contain the sodium urate crystal materials. Similar findings can be seen in other crystal deposition diseases or highly fibrotic lesions. A gouty nodule should be differentiated from nodules in rheumatoid arthritis.

ANATOMY AND PATHOLOGY OF THE FOOT

The foot has been divided traditionally into the hind-foot (calcaneus and talus), mid-foot (navicular, cuboid, and 3 cuneiforms), and forefoot (metatarsals and phalanges).[43] US assessment of

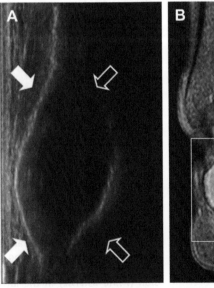
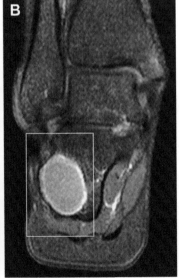

Fig. 23. (A) US image of an anechoic structure deep to the lateral cortex of the calcaneus. Although there is no through transmission in normal adult bone, thinning of the cortex (arrows) in this patient was sufficient to allow depiction of the deeper wall (arrow heads) of the simple bone cyst. The US image has been rotated to match the white box in Fig. 23B. (B) Correlative MR image of the calcaneus showing a simple bone cyst (inside box).

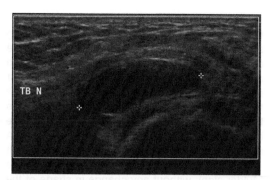

Fig. 24. US image of the tarsal tunnel showing a ganglion (marked with *calipers*) displacing the tibial nerve (TB N).

the tendons, joints, and soft tissue masses in the mid-foot and forefoot is mostly targeted on the area that is indicated by patients who have symptoms and discomfort.

The plantar plate (or plantar accessory ligament) is formed by fibers from the FHL, adductor hallucis, and abductor hallucis, which combine with the deep transverse metatarsal ligament to form a fibrocartilaginous plate along the plantar aspect of the metatarsophalangeal (MTP) joint capsule. The 2 sesamoids are contained within the plantar plate. This plate supports the metatarsal head and prevents hyperextension of the joint.[44]

Injury to the plantar plate can be delineated with high-resolution US.[45] It may be torn in women who wear high heels that shift the body's weight onto the hyperextended MTP joint. This stresses and stretches the plantar plate. The second MTP joint is the most vulnerable site for rupture. This is where

the plate is largest owing to the size of the second metatarsal bone. Associated hemorrhage, edema, synovitis, fluid within the flexor tendon, and sesamoid fracture may be demonstrated with US.

Sinus tarsi syndrome refers to a pain localized to the region of the sinus tarsi, most often related to traumatic rupture of the talocalcaneal ligament, or, less commonly, owing to inflammatory disease or foot deformity.[46]

Tarsal tunnel syndrome is caused by entrapment of the tibial nerve or its branches within the tarsal tunnel. The tunnel is a space made by medial surface of ankle and the overlying flexor retinaculum and contains the medial tendon group, as well as the neurovascular bundle and its branches. The syndrome is characterized by pain and paresthesia in the medial ankle radiating to the plantar aspect of the foot. The syndrome may be related to not only external compression by tight footwear or plaster casts but also intra-tunnel pathologies, such as ganglion (**Fig. 24**), osseous coalition, lipoma, varicose vein, accessory muscles, and intrinsic pathology of the nerve itself. US is effective in the identification of space-occupying lesions within the tunnel,[47] and in evaluation of abnormality of the tibial nerve.[48]

Foot disease in diabetes is multifactorial and results from a combination of peripheral angiopathy, peripheral neuropathy, and superimposed infection. MR has the advantage of quantification, precise localization, and evaluation of the extent of cellulitis, abscess, other fluid collection, osteomyelitis, sinus tract, neuropathy, and osseous involvement (**Fig. 25**A).[49] US of the diabetic foot, however, is better than MR in evaluation of

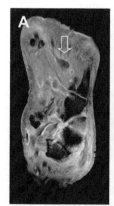

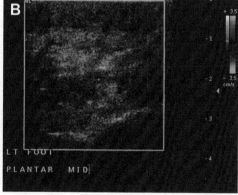

Fig. 25. (*A*) Contrast-enhanced T1 coronal image of the left foot showing rim enhancement around a structure (*empty arrow*) in the sole of the foot next to the plantar fascia. The lack of internal enhancement indicated that the contents are likely to be fluid and thus suspected of being an abscess. (*B*) Correlative US image of the sole of the foot showing that the structure has solid echogenic contents. It did not show a change in shape with grade compression and was though to represent an area of inflammation/phlegmon that had not liquefied. No drainage was performed as a result of the scan.

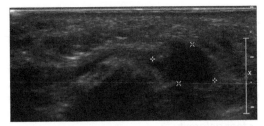

Fig. 26. US image of the sagittal plane between the second and third metatarsal from the dorsal side showing a hypoechoic ellipsoid Morton neuroma mass (between *calipers*). This is often palpable and painful on compression.

complicated tendinous and vascular pathology, although the role of US is still limited (see **Fig. 25B**). The thickness of plantar soft tissue may be decreased in a diabetic patient with ulceration.[50]

Masses and Tumors

A full discussion of soft tissue tumors is beyond the scope of this article; however, several items are mentioned in the following paragraphs.

Morton neuroma (or interdigital neuroma) is not a true neoplasm but rather a posttraumatic, degenerative, peri-neural fibrous mass of the plantar digital nerve at the level of the metatarsal head.[51] About 90% are in the second-third or third-fourth interdigital spaces. It is the most common nerve entrapment syndrome in the foot. About 80% of the patients affected are women (usually 25–50 years) and often there is bilateral involvement. It typically presents as a solid hypoechoic mass that is oval on axial, and ellipsoid on sagittal scans (**Fig. 26**).[52] There are two US techniques to differentiate Morton neuroma from interdigital bursitis in the forefoot. The first is application of pressure with the examiner's finger

tip on the plantar aspect to splay out the intermetatarsal distance opposite the dorsal surface being scanned by a transducer placed transversely. The other is the sonographic Mulder test in which a transducer is placed transversely in the plantar aspect in the metatarsal head level with application of opposed medial-lateral stress to compress the metatarsal heads with the examiner's free hand on the dorsal aspect of the forefoot. A neuroma is displaced to the plantar aspect with a jerk movement and a palpable click (the positive Mulder sign), without any change in shape of the mass. However, interdigital bursitis shows fluid-filled space that is easily compressible and changeable in contour (**Fig. 27**).[53] Neuromas are commonly found with bursitis.

Traumatic (or amputation stump) neuroma occurs when a nerve is severed. Stump pain is a frequent presentation and may be related to abnormal electrical activity. The US finding, although nonspecific, is that of hypoechoic mass with irregular or poorly defined margin.[54] US can serve as a guide for a needle biopsy.

Foreign bodies can be easily diagnosed with US, especially for detecting radiolucent bodies on radiography, including glass, wood, metal, cotton ball, and so on. Foreign bodies can be detected both by the echoes they produce and their effect on the distal sound beam; depending on their size, glass and wood fragments may shadow,[55] and metal objects tend to produce comet-tail reverberation artifact (**Fig. 28**). A hypoechoic inflammatory halo can often be seen around foreign bodies.[56] Once found, marking on the skin over the foreign body is helpful for subsequent removal. The size, extent, and the relationship with adjacent vascular/nervous structures can be evaluated.

Painful bone diseases can be detected on US even without a history of acute trauma.[57] Stress

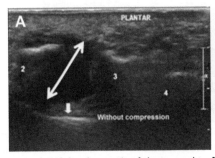
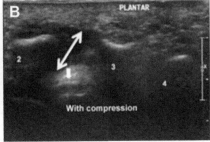

Fig. 27. (*A*) US image of the short axis of the second to fourth metatarsal bones showing a bursa (*double headed arrow*) at the second interdigital web space (between the second and third metatarsal heads). This is round when not compressed. (*B*) When compressed with the examiner's finger (*white arrow*), there is an alteration of the size and shape of the bursa.

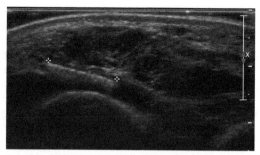

Fig. 28. US image of the coronal plane in the lateral aspect of the calcaneus and cuboid bone. A linear hyperechoic metallic foreign body is present (marked with *calipers*) that shows reverberation artifacts. It was confirmed as a broken sewing needle at surgery.

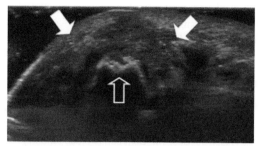

Fig. 30. US image of the ankle in a patient with chronic pain after removal of a screw placed in the medial malleolus for internal fixation of a fracture. A hypoechoic soft tissue mass (*white arrow*) is present around the cortical irregularity of the medial malleolus (*arrow head*). Fibrotic tissue and inflammatory hyperplasia was excised from the screw removal site.

fractures are most common at the second or third metatarsal bones. The US findings of stress fracture are disrupted cortex, step-off deformity, focally thick hyperechoic line representing periosteal reaction, and curved hyperechoic callus overlying the cortical interruption (**Fig. 29**).[58] Understanding of US findings of fractures will heighten the perception of bone abnormalities that are incidentally found during scanning.[59]

Postoperative Conditions

Radiography cannot visualize soft tissue abnormality in patients with orthopedic metallic hardware. Computed tomography and MRI are also usually inadequate because of image degradation by metallic artifacts. US may useful in identifying and depicting hardware-related soft tissue complications, such as hematoma, abscess, seroma, impingement, and osseous complication (**Fig. 30**).[60]

SUMMARY

With US, tendon and ligament diseases are easily diagnosed and distinguished from other periarticular and intra-articular diseases in the ankle. US is highly useful when a dynamic examination is performed in cases in which physical examination is limited. Thus, US is a rapid and cost-effective diagnostic tool for problem solving in the ankle and foot.

REFERENCES

1. Jacobson JA. Introduction to musculoskeletal ultrasound. Ultrasound Clin 2007;2:569–76. http://dx.doi.org/10.1016/j.cult.2008.01.005.
2. Finlay K, Friedman L. Ultrasonography of the lower extremity. Orthop Clin North Am 2006;37:245–75.
3. Fananapazir G, Allison SJ. Common applications of musculoskeletal ultrasound in the emergency department. Ultrasound Clin 2011;6:215–26.
4. De Maeseneer M, Marcelis S, Jager T, et al. Sonography of the normal ankle: a target approach using skeletal reference points. Am J Roentgenol 2009;192:487–95.
5. Doral MN, Alam M, Bozkurt M, et al. Functional anatomy of the Achilles tendon. Knee Surg Sports Traumatol Arthrosc 2010;18(5):638–43.
6. Pang BS, Ying M. Sonographic measurement of Achilles tendons in asymptomatic subjects: variation with age, body height, and dominance of ankle. J Ultrasound Med 2006;25(10):1291–6.
7. Szaro P, Witkowski G, Smigielski R, et al. Fascicles of the adult human Achilles tendon—anatomical study. Annals Ana 2009;191:586–93.
8. O'Brien M. The anatomy of the Achilles tendon. Foot Ankle Clin 2005;10(2):225–38.
9. Hatzantonis C, Agur A, Naraghi A, et al. Dissecting the accessory soleus muscle: a literature review,

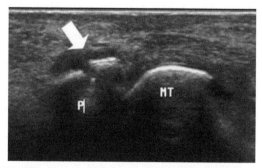

Fig. 29. US image of the sagittal plane showing the head of the second metatarsal bone (MT) and proximal phalanx (P) in the plantar aspect. There is a fracture at the base of the proximal phalanx (*white arrow*) of the second toe.

cadaveric study, and imaging study. Clin Anat 2011; 24(7):903–10.

10. Thompson J, Baravarian B. Acute and chronic Achilles tendon ruptures in athletes. Clin Podiatr Med Surg 2011;28(1):117–35.

11. Hartgerink P, Fessell DP, Jacobson JA, et al. Full- versus partial-thickness Achilles tendon tears: sono- graphic accuracy and characterization in 26 cases with surgical correlation. Radiology 2001;220:406–12.

12. Wilson JJ, Best TM. Common overuse tendon prob- lems: a review and recommendations for treatment. Am Fam Physician 2005;72(5):811–8.

13. Järvinen TA, Kannus P, Maffulli N, et al. Achilles tendon disorders: etiology and epidemiology. Foot Ankle Clin 2005;10(2):255–66.

14. Khan KM, Cool JL, Kannus P, et al. Time to abandon the "tendinitis" myth. BMJ 2002;324(7338):626–7.

15. Paavola M, Kannus P, Jarvinen TA, et al. Achilles ten- dinopathy. J Bone Joint Surg Am 2002;84:2062–76.

16. Nehrer S, Breitenseher M, Brodner W, et al. Clinical and sonographic evaluation of the risk of rupture in the Achilles tendon. Arch Orthop Trauma Surg 1997;116(1–2):14–8.

17. Schepsis AA, Jones H, Haas AL. Achilles tendon disorders in athletes. Am J Sports Med 2002;30(2): 287–305.

18. Van Dijk CN, van Sterkenburg MN, Wiegerinck JI, et al. Terminology for Achilles tendon related disor- ders. Knee Surg Sports Traumatol Arthrosc 2011; 19(5):835–41.

19. Kvist M, Jozsa L, Jarvinen MJ, et al. Chronic Achilles paratenonitis in athletes: a histological and histo- chemical study. Pathology 1987;19:1–11.

20. Pavlov H, Heneghan MA, Hersh A, et al. The Ha- glund syndrome: initial and differential diagnosis. Radiology 1982;144(1):83–8.

21. Schweitzer ME, Leersum M, Ehrlich SS, et al. Fluid in normal and abnormal ankle joints: amount and distri- bution as seen on MR images. Am J Roentgenol 1994;162:111–4.

22. Nazarian LN, Rawool NM, Martin CE, et al. Synovial fluid in the hindfoot and ankle: detection of amount and distribution with US. Radiology 1995;197:275–8.

23. Negrine JP. Tibialis anterior rupture: acute and chronic. Foot Ankle Clin 2007;12(4):569–72.

24. Thomas JL, Lopez-Ben R, Maddox J. A preliminary report on intra-sheath peroneal tendon subluxation: a prospective review of 7 patients with ultrasound verification. J Foot Ankle Surg 2009;48(3):323–9.

25. Ebraheim NA, Taser F, Shafig Q, et al. Anatomical evaluation and clinical importance of the tibiofibular syndesmosis ligaments. Surg Radiol Anat 2006;28: 142–9.

26. Schepers T. Acute distal tibiofibular syndesmosis injury: a systematic review of suture-button versus syndesmotic screw repair. Int Orthop 2012;36(6): 1199–206.

27. Taser F, Shafig Q, Ebraheim NA. Anatomy of lateral ankle ligaments and their relationship to bony land- marks. Surg Radiol Anat 2006;28:391–7.

28. Oae K, Takao M, Uchio Y, et al. Evaluation of anterior talofibular ligament injury with stress radiography, ultrasonography and MR imaging. Skeletal Radiol 2010;39:41–7.

29. Ferran NA, Maffulli N. Epidemiology of sprains of the lateral ankle ligament complex. Foot Ankle Clin 2006;11(3):659–62.

30. Ivins D. Acute ankle sprain: an update. Am Fam Physician 2006;74(10):1714–20.

31. Mansour R, Jibri Z, Kamath S, et al. Persistent ankle pain following a sprain: a review of imaging. Emerg Radiol 2011;18:211–25.

32. Nallamshetty L, Nazarian LN, Schweitzer ME, et al. Evaluation of posterior tibial pathology: comparison of sonography and MR imaging. Skeletal Radiol 2005;34(7):375–80.

33. Khan K, Brown J, Way S, et al. Overuse injuries in classical ballet. Sports Med 1995;19(5):341–57.

34. McMillan AM, Landorf KB, Barrett JT, et al. Diag- nostic imaging for chronic plantar heel pain: a systematic review and meta-analysis. J Foot Ankle Res 2009;2:32.

35. Griffith JF, Wong TY, Wong SM, et al. Sonography of plantar fibromatosis. Am J Roentgenol 2002;179(5): 1167–72.

36. Melchiorre D, Linari S, Innocenti M, et al. Ultrasound detects joint damage and bleeding in haemophilic arthropathy: a proposal of a score. Haemophilia 2011;17(1):112–7.

37. Janow GL, Panghaal V, Trinh A, et al. Detection of active disease in juvenile idiopathic arthritis: sensi- tivity and specificity of the physical examination vs ultrasound. J Rheumatol 2011;38(12):2671–4.

38. Chen YC, Hsu SW. Tuberculous arthritis mimic arthritis of the Sjögren's syndrome: findings from sonography, computed tomography and mag- netic resonance images. Eur J Radiol 2001; 40(3):232–5.

39. McCarthy CL, Wilson DJ, Coltman TP. Anterolateral ankle impingement: findings and diagnostic accu- racy with ultrasound imaging. Skeletal Radiol 2008; 37:209–16.

40. Bianchi S, Martinoli C. Detection of loose bodies in joints. Radiol Clin North Am 1999;37(4):679–90.

41. Frankel DA, Bargiela A, Bouffard JA, et al. Synovial joints: evaluation of intraarticular bodies with US. Radiology 1998;206(1):41–4.

42. Filippucci E, Meenagh G, Delle Sedie A, et al. Ultra- sound imaging for the rheumatologist XXXVI. Sono- graphic assessment of the foot in gout patients. Clin Exp Rheumatol 2011;29(6):901–5.

43. Ansede G, Lee JC, Healy JC. Musculoskeletal sonography of the normal foot. Skeletal Radiol 2010;39:225–42.

44. Yao L, Do HM, Cracchiolo A, et al. Plantar plate of the foot: findings on conventional arthrography and MR imaging. Am J Roentgenol 1994;163(3):641–4.

45. Khoury V, Guillin R, Dhanju J, et al. Ultrasound of ankle and foot: overuse and sports injuries. Semin Musculoskelet Radiol 2007;11(2):149–61.

46. Helgeson K. Examination and intervention for sinus tarsi syndrome. N Am J Sports Phys Ther 2009; 4(1):29–37.

47. Fantino O, Coillard JY, Borne J, et al. Ultrasound of the tarsal tunnel: normal and pathological imaging features. J Radiol 2011;92(12):1072–80.

48. Kotnis N, Harish S, Popowich T. Medial ankle and heel: ultrasound evaluation and sonographic appearances of conditions causing symptoms. Semin Ultrasound CT MR 2011;32:125–41.

49. Loredo R, Rahal A, Garcia G, et al. Imaging of the diabetic foot: diagnostic dilemmas. Foot Ankle Spec 2010;3(5):249–64.

50. Abouaesha F, van Schie CH, Griffths GD, et al. Plantar tissue thickness is related to peak plantar pressure in the high-risk diabetic foot. Diabetes Care 2001;24(7):1270–4.

51. Mulder JD. The causative mechanisms in Morton's metatarsalgia. J Bone Joint Surg Br 1951;33:94–5.

52. Lee MJ, Kim S, Huh YM, et al. Morton neuroma: evaluated with ultrasonography and MR imaging. Korean J Radiol 2007;8(2):148–55.

53. Torriani M, Kattapuram SV. Dynamic sonography of the forefoot: the sonographic Mulder sign. Am J Roentgenol 2003;180:1121–3.

54. Provost N, Bonaldi VM, Sarazin L, et al. Amputation stump neuroma: ultrasound features. J Clin Ultrasound 1997;25(2):85–9.

55. Shrestha D, Sharma UK, Mohammad R, et al. The role of ultrasonography in detection and localization of radiolucent foreign body in soft tissues of extremities. JNMA J Nepal Med Assoc 2009; 48(173):5–9.

56. Horton LK, Jacobson JA, Powell A, et al. Sonography and radiography of soft-tissue foreign bodies. Am J Roentgenol 2001;176(5):1155–9.

57. Cho KH, Lee SM, Lee YH, et al. Ultrasound diagnosis of either an occult or missed fracture of an extremity in pediatric-aged children. Korean J Radiol 2010;11:84–94.

58. Banal F, Gandjbakhch F, Foltz V, et al. Sensitivity and specificity of ultrasonography in early diagnosis of metatarsal bone stress fractures: a pilot study of 37 patients. J Rheumatol 2009;36(8):1715–9.

59. Cho KH, Lee YH, Lee SM, et al. Sonography of bone and bone-related diseases of the extremities. J Clin Ultrasound 2004;32:511–21.

60. Guillin R, Bianchi S. Sonographic assessment of orthopedic hardware impingement on soft tissues of the limbs. J Ultrasound 2012;15:50–5.

Sonography of Cutaneous and Ungual Lumps and Bumps

Ximena Wortsman, MD

KEYWORDS

- Skin ultrasound • Ultrasound dermatology • Skin imaging • Cutaneous sonography
- Nail ultrasound • Nail sonography • Skin cancer • Cutaneous tumors

KEY POINTS

- Ultrasonography provides anatomic information in common cutaneous and ungual conditions.
- Measurements in all axes, including depth, as well as the echostructure and vascularity patterns of the lesions may support the diagnosis and the medical and surgical management.
- Discrimination of the dermatologic and nondermatologic origin of the conditions can also be possible.

INTRODUCTION

Cutaneous and ungual applications of sonography have been increasing in recent years, mostly related to the development of a new generation of ultrasound machines that have probes with higher variable frequencies, more channels, and color Doppler sensitivity. Thus, this more sophisticated equipment give us reasonable resolution for identifying the skin layers and deeper structures without losing definition when changing the focal region of study.[1] Additionally, patients and physicians are demanding information about anatomic data that can support an early diagnosis and adequate management as well as improve the cosmetic result in dermatologic entities.

The skin is the largest organ in the body and is a complex structure where multiple physiologic processes take place. It is both our visible presentation to society and an efficient defensive organ to the hostile external environment. Thus, any injury to the skin can affect our quality of life or self-esteem.[2,3]

On the other hand, the nail is an integral part of the digital tip and a complex enthesis where the ungual and periungual tissues are closely interconnected with the joint, ligaments, capsule, and tendinous structures. The nail is also an organ that responds to systemic changes.[4] Biopsies of the nail can be difficult to perform, however, and

may leave cosmetic sequels. This may favor the usage of imaging techniques in this structure.[5,6]

Both the skin and nail may be affected by various primary and secondary conditions. These latter are generated in neighboring structures, such as muscle, cartilage, or bone and secondarily involve the skin or ungual regions.

Sonography has many advantages for studying the skin and nail, among them are a suitable balance between resolution and penetration, and a real-time provision of anatomic information, which includes the assessment of the characteristics of blood flow, the lack of radiation effects, or confinement of the patient in a reduced space. Limitations of this technique are few and currently include epidermal-only lesions, or those that measure less than 0.1 mm, and the detection of pigments, including melanin.[1] However, small calcium deposits and fragments of hair can be easily identified.

Thus, owing to the high sensitivity of the color Doppler in the new generation of machines, contrast medium is rarely used in baseline cutaneous sonographic studies; this may prevent the potential development of adverse reactions. During the examinations, moreover, there is a full, live interaction between the patient and the sonographer that allows the correlation of the visible dermatologic

Department of Radiology and Department of Dermatology, Clinica Servet, Faculty of Medicine, University of Chile, Almirante Pastene 150, Santiago, Chile
E-mail address: xwo@tie.cl

Ultrasound Clin 7 (2012) 505–523
http://dx.doi.org/10.1016/j.cult.2012.08.006
1556-858X/12/$ – see front matter © 2012 Elsevier Inc. All rights reserved.

findings with the sonographic images on the screen. Furthermore, the sonographer can make immediate decisions in vivo, such as whether to include another body region not primarily requested.[3]

The aim of this article was to review the potential of sonography in common dermatologic lesions that may clinically show as lumps or bumps in the skin or nail.

TECHNICAL CONSIDERATIONS

It is recommended that this type of examination should be performed with multichannel machines and variable frequency probes that reach frequencies of 15 MHz or higher. The latter comment does not detract from the use of lower frequencies but commonly the definition of the skin layers improves at higher frequencies. Usually, compact linear probes (hockey stick type) adapt better to the concavities and convexities of the cutaneous or nail surface, which may be important, for example in the face, or when dealing with lesions in small corporal segments, such as the fingers. Nevertheless, wider linear probes are also used in large-size lesions to cover the whole extent of the abnormalities or when comparing normal versus abnormal tissues.

Extended field of view, compound software, and 3-dimensional reconstructions, as well as sensitive color Doppler capabilities, may facilitate the provision and understanding of information by the clinician.

After a visual inspection of the lesion(s) the sonographer applies a copious amount of gel to the skin or nail surface. Commonly, no stand-off pads are required; furthermore, any potential compression of the skin vessels should be avoided.

Nails are examined with the finger or toe fully extended. If necessary, a pad or towel can be used to support the thumbs. A gray-scale and color Doppler sweep that includes at least 2 perpendicular axes is then performed.

For better definition of the hair follicles in the scalp, it is recommended to avoid softening softwares (ie, median filtering) and to displace the hair tracts from the area of the lesion.

Sedation is used in our department on children younger than 4 years to avoid artifacts derived from crying or moving. We use chloral hydrate (50 mg/kg) orally administered 30 minutes before the examination and after an informed consent is signed by the parent or guardian. The modified Aldrete score may be used to monitor the children during the sedation process. This score includes the evaluation of activity, respiration, circulation (blood pressure), consciousness, and oxygen saturation. Nine or more points are used to discharge the patient.

The settings include power Doppler to detect slow-flow, low-pulse repetition frequencies and wall filters, and a color gain below the noise threshold to acquire high-quality images.

Three-dimensional reconstructions are commonly performed by making 5-second to 8-second sweeps within the area of the lesion, to highlight the presentation of the lesion.[1,3]

NORMAL SONOGRAPHIC ANATOMY OF THE SKIN, NAIL, AND HAIR

Anatomically, the skin presents 3 layers: epidermis, dermis, and hypodermis, also called subcutaneous tissue. These layers are closely connected, and many of the pathologic conditions may involve more than one layer. The echogenicity of the cutaneous layers depends on their main components. For example, the echogenicity of the epidermis is a result of the high content of keratin; in the dermis, it depends on the collagen content and in the hypodermis, the echogenicity is a result of the fatty tissue. On sonography, the epidermis appears as a bright hyperechoic line in nonglabrous skin (all but the palms and soles) and as a bilaminar parallel hyperechoic structure in the palmar and plantar skin. The dermis shows as a hyperechoic band; however, less bright than the epidermis. Nevertheless, because of the damage produced by UV radiation over time, a deposit of glycosaminoglycans, also called elastosis, may be shown in the upper dermis, which can be detected on ultrasound as a subepidermal low-echogenicity band. The hypodermis presents hypoechogenicity, owing to fatty lobules, with hyperechoic fibrous septa in between. On color Doppler, low-flow arterial and venous vessels are detected in the hypodermis but rarely in the dermis (**Fig. 1**).[3]

The nail presents 2 main parts: the ungual and periungual regions. The ungual part is composed of the nail bed (which includes the matrix region) and the nail plate. The periungual tissue is composed of the lateral and proximal nail folds, as well as the bony margin of the distal phalanx. On sonography, the nail bed appears hypoechoic, and occasionally turns to slightly hyperechoic in the proximal region underneath the ungual matrix. The nail plate appears as a bilaminar structure made up of 2 hyperechoic, parallel lines called the dorsal (dp) and ventral (vp) plates. The origin of the nail plate is usually distal to the level of the distal interphalangeal joint. The proximal and lateral nail folds present the same cutaneous echostructure as the rest of the body, but mostly

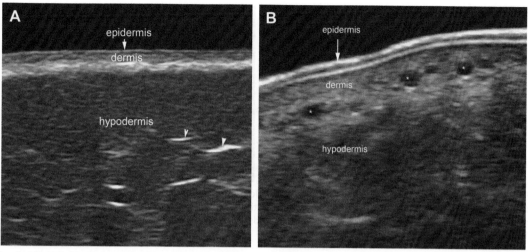

Fig. 1. Normal skin (gray-scale ultrasound). (*A*) Normal nonglabrous skin (transverse view, ventral left arm) shows the cutaneous layers: epidermis, dermis, and hypodermis. The small arrowheads are pointing out the normal hyperechoic fibrous septa at the hypodermis. (*B*) Normal glabrous skin at the plantar region (transverse view) demonstrates the typical bilaminar hyperechoic pattern of the glabrous epidermis. Venous vessels (*asterisk*) in the upper hypodermis are also detected.

lack fatty tissue. The bony margin of the distal phalanx shows as a hyperechoic line underneath the nail bed. Commonly, slow-flow arterial and venous vessels are detected in the nail bed (**Fig. 2**).[6]

The hair is composed of 2 main regions: the hair follicle (located in the dermis) and the hair tract (the visible part). The hair follicles show as dermal hypoechoic bands with oblique disposition (**Fig. 3**). The axes and density of the hair follicles may change according to ethnic factors or anatomic regions. The hair tracts located on the scalp show a trilaminar hyperechoic appearance owing to the keratin content and their disposition. The 2 outer layers compose the cuticle-cortex complex and the inner layer corresponds to the medulla (**Fig. 4**). The villous hair located in the rest of the body appears on sonography as a hyperechoic monolaminar structure. The latter appearance includes the eyelashes and the hair of the eyebrows.[7]

PATHOLOGY
Cutaneous Tumors and Pseudotumors

Benign conditions
Cysts
Epidermal cyst These cysts originate in epidermal components that are abnormally located in the dermis and hypodermis. Clinically, epidermal cysts show as skin-colored or erythematous lumps that may discharge oily or cheesy material. On histology, they are composed of stratified squamous epithelium with a granular layer but without a sebaceous basis. Thus, "sebaceous cyst" is a misnomer and should not be used. On sonography, they can vary in their appearance according to the phase of the cyst. Hence, intact epidermal

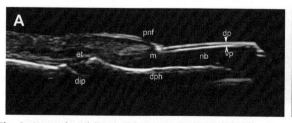
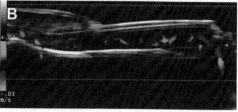

Fig. 2. Normal nail (longitudinal view). (*A*) Gray-scale ultrasound shows the different parts of the nail unit. (*B*) Color Doppler ultrasound demonstrates the normal blood flow within the nail bed. nb, nail bed; dp, dorsal plate; vp, ventral plate; m, matrix; pnf, proximal nail fold; dph, distal phalanx; dip, distal interphalangeal joint; et, extensor tendon insertion (distal part of the lateral slips).

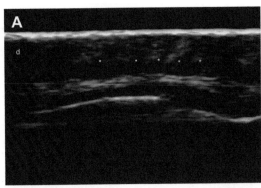 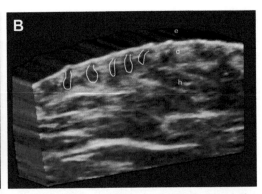

Fig. 3. Normal hair follicles. (*A*) Gray-scale ultrasound (longitudinal view at the scalp-occipital region) shows several hypoechoic oblique bands that correspond to the hair follicles (*asterisks*) in the dermis. (*B*) Three-dimensional reconstruction (longitudinal view, 5–8 seconds sweep, left axilla) demonstrates the hair follicles outlined. d, dermis; e, epidermis; h, hypodermis.

cysts are shown as round-shaped, well-defined, anechoic structures in the dermis and hypodermis that may also present a thin anechoic tract connecting them to the subepidermal region, called "punctum." When the cyst becomes inflamed, however, it can show a pseudosolid and heterogeneous giant structure sometimes presenting a "pseudotestes appearance" (ie, brighter inner echoes and anechoic filiform areas). If a rupture of the cyst occurs, the release of keratin to the surrounding tissue generates a foreign-body–like inflammatory reaction and the cyst can be shown as an irregular or lobulated hypoechoic pseudosolid lesion. Usually, during all the phases, a posterior acoustic enhancement artifact shown by the cyst is conserved, which may facilitate diagnosis. On color Doppler examination, increased vascularity with thin, slow-flow vessels may be detected in the periphery of the cyst mostly during the inflammation and rupture stages (**Figs. 5 and 6**).[3,8,9]

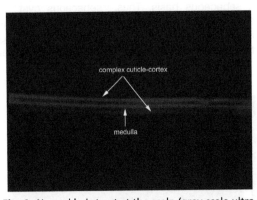

Fig. 4. Normal hair tract at the scalp (gray-scale ultrasound, longitudinal view). Notice the trilaminar hyperechoic appearance of the hair tract with an outer complex cuticle–cortex and the medulla in the center of the structure.

Trichilemmal cyst Clinically, trichilemmal cysts appear as single or multiple skin-colored or erythematous firm swellings or nodules, commonly associated with focal baldness, because their main location is the scalp. Also called pilar cysts, they are derived from the external sheath of the hair follicle and are lined with cuboidal epidermal cells. In contrast to epidermal cysts, trichilemmal cysts do not contain a granular layer and commonly do not show a tract connecting to the subepidermal region (punctum). They contain compact keratin, and sometimes hair fragments and oily material that may be prone to calcification. On sonography, trichilemmal cysts show as round-shaped, well-defined, anechoic or hypoechoic structures located in the dermis and hypodermis, that may occasionally demonstrate inner echoes (debris), hyperechoic spots of calcium deposits, or hyperechoic lines that correspond to hair fragments. Posterior acoustic transmission is usually conserved especially in the noncalcified trichilemmal cysts. The presence of calcium deposits within a trichilemmal cyst may mimic the sonographic appearance of pilomatrixoma, a benign tumor derived from the hair matrix. Nevertheless, in contrast to pilomatrixomas, these cysts usually show a thick rim and lack of vascularity. On color Doppler examination, they are usually hypovascular, although with inflammation, trichilemmal cysts may show peripheral vascularity with slow-flow vessels (**Fig. 7**).[7,10]

Pilonidal cyst These cysts frequently affect young adults and are located in the intergluteal region. Pilonidal cysts originate with the embedding of hair tracts within the skin layers, through dilated follicular ostia. Chronic regional trauma from continuous friction, excessive body hair, obesity, or occupations requiring sitting, are reported among the causes.

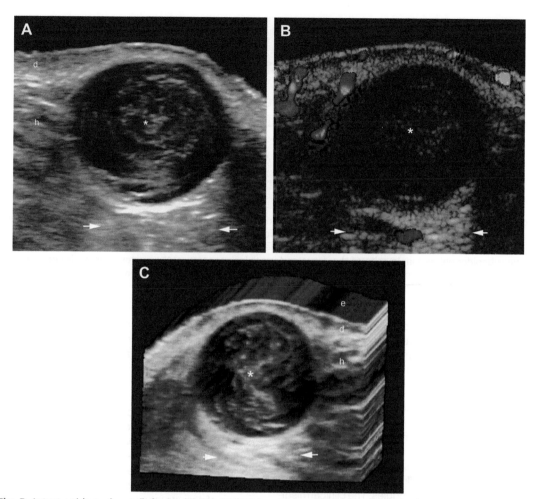

Fig. 5. Intact epidermal cyst (left cheek). (*A*) Gray-scale ultrasound (*longitudinal view*) shows a round-shaped, well-defined, hypoechoic structure (*asterisk*) located in the upper hypodermis and dermis. The lesion presents some filiform anechoic areas and posterior acoustic enhancement (*arrows*). (*B*) Color Doppler ultrasound (*longitudinal view*) shows increased vascularity in the periphery of the lesion compatible with inflammatory changes. (*C*) Three-dimensional reconstruction (5–8 seconds sweep, *longitudinal view*) that highlights the cyst (*asterisk*). Notice the posterior acoustic enhancement (*arrows*). d, dermis; e, epidermis; h, hypodermis.

These pseudocystic structures or sinuses contain a nest of hair tracts and keratin and can easily become inflamed and/or infected, thus, they can show as an erythematous swelling that drains oily or purulent material.

On sonography, they appear as oval-shaped, well-defined anechoic or hypoechoic structures in the dermis, and subcutaneous tissue with hyperechoic lines that correspond to the hair tracts. Moreover, the axis of the cyst and its branches may be sonographically assessed. On color Doppler examination, increased vascularity may be detected in the periphery of the cysts (**Fig. 8**).[3,11]

Solid lesions

Lipomatous tumors Lipomatous tumors are the most common soft tissue tumors and are composed of mature adipose cells, usually mixed with fibrous (fibrolipoma) or capillary (angiolipoma) components. Lipomas can show as single or multiple, painless, and firm lumps, although rarely they may show tenderness on extrinsic compression of the surrounding structures. On sonography, lipomas are shown as well-defined oval-shaped structures in the hypodermis that follow the axis of the cutaneous layers. Fibrolipomas commonly appear as hypoechoic, and angiolipomas appear hyperechoic and/or heterogeneous.[12–14] Interspersed within the tissue there are hyperechoic fibrous septa, usually more evident in the fibrolipoma type (**Fig. 9**). On color Doppler examination, they are frequently hypovascular, although any focal hypervascularity may suggest an atypical or neoplastic transformation. Sonography may be useful to provide the exact

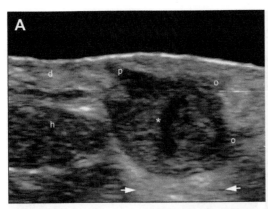
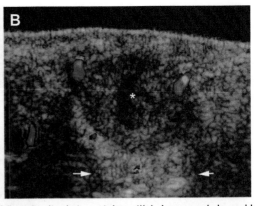

Fig. 6. Ruptured epidermal cyst. (A) Gray-scale ultrasound (longitudinal view, right axilla) shows oval-shaped hypoechoic structure (*asterisk*) located in the upper hypodermis and dermis with a central hypoechoic band. Notice the protrusions of hypoechoic material (keratin) into the surrounding tissue (o) and the connecting punctum (p) to the subepidermal region. In spite of the dense and irregular appearance, the posterior acoustic enhancement is conserved (*arrows*). (B) Color Doppler ultrasound (longitudinal view, right axilla) demonstrates increased vascularity in the periphery of the lesion (*asterisk*). d, dermis; h, hypodermis.

location of lipomas that occasionally can present risky locations close to large-size vessels, nerves, or glands. This is even more relevant in anatomic locations where the skin is thin, such as in the face, neck, and ventral forearm.

Pilomatrixoma Pilomatrixomas are benign tumors, also called pilomatricomas or calcifying epitheliomas of Malherbe, that originate in the hair matrix. Clinically, pilomatrixomas are commonly present in children and young adults and appear as single or multiple, slow-growing, firm to hard, skin-colored, erythematosus, or bluish nodules. The clinical misdiagnosis rate is high, and has been reported as up to 56% of the cases.[15] Therefore, pilomatrixomas may

easily simulate other common dermatologic entities, such as epidermal cysts. On histology, they are made up of lobules with basal and ghost cells, eosinophilic keratinous debris, and calcifications surrounded by a fibrous pseudocapsule of connective tissue.

On sonography, the typical appearance is a target lesion that shows as a round-shaped or lobulated nodule, with hypoechoic rim and hyperechoic center, located in the dermis and hypodermis. In 68% to 80% of the cases, hyperechoic spots that correspond to calcium deposits are detected in the center of the structure and compose one of the key sonographic elements for diagnosing a pilomatrixoma (**Fig. 10**).[16–18] Rarely, a cystic variant of

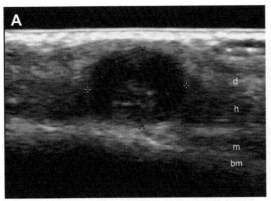
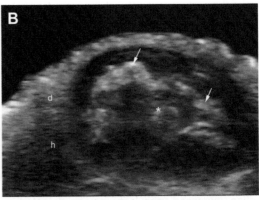

Fig. 7. Trichilemmal cyst. (A) Gray-scale ultrasound (left parietal region of the scalp) shows round-shaped, well-defined anechoic cystic structure (between markers) with some hypoechoic echoes (debris), located in the dermis and hypodermis. (B) Gray-scale ultrasound in other patient (left parietal region of the scalp) demonstrates a round-shaped well-defined structure with hypoechoic rim and heterogeneous center (*asterisk*) with some hyperechoic deposits (*arrows*) that correspond to dystrophic calcifications and hair fragments. bm; bony margin of the skull; d, dermis; h, hypodermis; m, epicranius muscle.

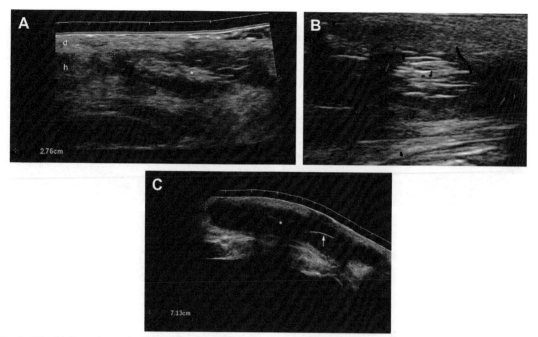

Fig. 8. Pilonidal cyst (intergluteal region). (*A*) Gray-scale ultrasound (*longitudinal view*) shows 2.76-cm-long, well-defined, oval-shaped, hypoechoic structure that involves dermis and hypodermis and presents hyperechoic lines that correspond to hair fragments (*asterisk*). (*B*) Power Doppler ultrasound (*longitudinal view*) demonstrates increased vascularity in the periphery of the lesion. Notice the prominent hyperechogenicity of the hair tracts within the structure. (*C*) Gray-scale ultrasound (*extended field of view, longitudinal axis*) shows 7.13-cm-long, well-defined, oval-shaped and hypoechoic structure (*asterisk*) located in the dermis and hypodermis. A hair fragment (*arrow*) is also pointed out.

pilomatrixomas can be detected, and shows on sonography as a mixed solid-cystic structure with a thick hypoechoic wall, anechoic fluid, sometimes with echoes and septa, as well as a hypoechoic nodular solid part with variable degrees of hyperechoic calcium deposits. The latter appearance is usually caused by hemorrhage episodes within the pilomatrixoma, and may clinically cause a fast growing erythematous lesion that can be clinically mistaken for a malignant and/or vascular tumor. On color Doppler examination, these benign entities can show variable vascularity that can go from hypovascular to hypervascular, usually with slow-flow, thin vessels both in the center and the rim. Moreover,

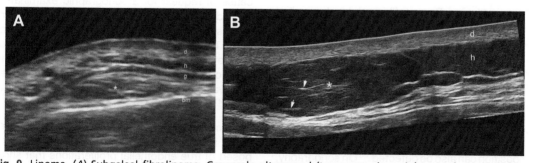

Fig. 9. Lipoma. (*A*) Subgaleal fibrolipoma. Gray-scale ultrasound (transverse view, right temple region) shows a subgaleal, oval-shaped, well-defined hypoechoic nodule (*asterisk*) following the axis of the skin layers and located between the epicranius muscle (galea, g) and the bony margin of the skull. Some hyperechoic fibrous septa are also possible to define within the nodule. (*B*) Giant fibrolipoma. Gray scale (longitudinal view, right lumbar region) demonstrates a well-defined, oval-shaped large hypoechoic structure (*) in the hypodermis that follows the axis of the cutaneous layers and presents hyperechoic septa (*arrows*). bm, bony margin of the skull; d, dermis; h, hypodermis; g, galea.

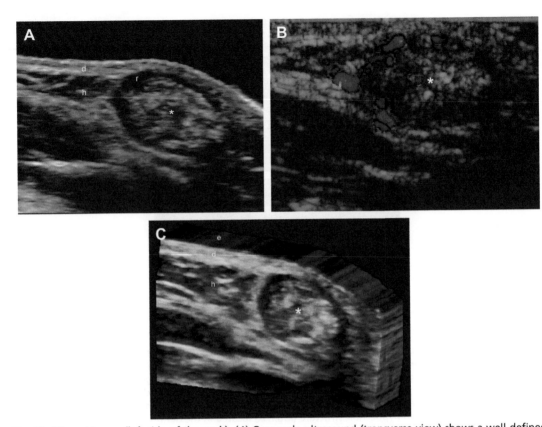

Fig. 10. Pilomatrixoma (left side of the neck). (*A*) Gray-scale ultrasound (transverse view) shows a well-defined, round-shaped nodule with hypoechoic rim (r) and hyperechoic center (*asterisk*) that affects dermis and hypodermis. The tiny hyperechoic spots in the center of the lesion correspond to small deposits of calcium. (*B*) Color Doppler ultrasound (transverse view) demonstrates slightly increased vascularity mostly in the periphery of the nodule (*asterisk*). (*C*) Three-dimensional reconstruction (5–8 seconds sweep) of the lesion (*). e, epidermis; d, dermis; h, hypodermis; r, rim.

there are reports of hypervascular pilomatrixomas that can clinically mimic a hemangioma.[19] In these cases, the sonographic support may be of paramount importance.

Dermatofibroma Dermatofibroma is also called fibrous histiocytoma, or histiocytoma cutis. Clinically, dermatofibromas commonly show as a slow-growing, erythematous or brown, firm, painless nodule in the lower extremities or trunk of middle-aged women. They are thought to be reactive lesions related to trauma or insect bites. On histology, they show spindle cells and a hyaline collagenous stroma. Scattered lipid-laden histiocytes, multinucleated giant cells, and hemosiderin deposition can also be detected.[20] On sonography, dermatofibromas show as an ill-defined hypoechoic and heterogeneous structure that affects the dermis but may also extend to the upper hypodermis and can be associated with a distortion or enlargement of the local hair follicles in the dermis (**Fig. 11**). On color Doppler examination, they are

commonly hypovascular but may also show prominent vascularity with thin, slow-flow vessels.

Vascular lesions Vascular lesions are a common cause of request for a sonographic examination in children and babies. The most frequent vascular lesions are hemangiomas and vascular malformations. This separation is based on the clinical findings, evolution, and histologic characteristics and prognosis of these 2 types of vascular anomalies and was proposed by Mulliken and Glowacki in 1982.[21]

Hemangiomas Hemangiomas are the most frequent soft tissue tumor in infancy and are composed of true endothelial proliferations that show rapid growth after birth, followed by a plateau after 2 or 3 years and then a slow regression phase that may last 5 or 6 years. In contrast, vascular malformations are errors in morphogenesis composed of a disproportionately high number of vascular channels that grow proportionally with the child.

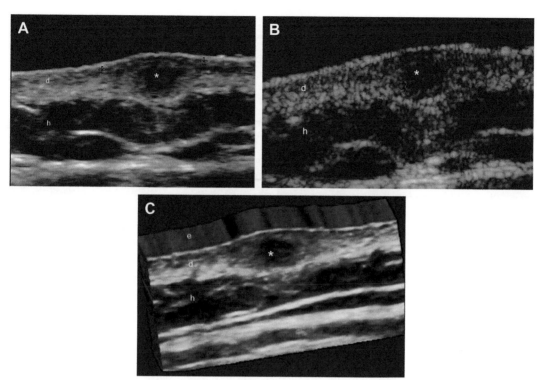

Fig. 11. Dermatofibroma (left dorsal region). (*A*) Gray-scale ultrasound (transverse view) shows ill-defined hypoechoic fusiform dermal structure (*asterisk*, between markers). (*B*) Color Doppler ultrasound demonstrates small vessels in the periphery of the lesion. (*C*) Three-dimensional reconstruction (5–8 seconds sweep) of the lesional area (*). e, epidermis; d, dermis; h, hypodermis.

According to the type of channel, they can be subdivided into arterial, venous, lymphatic, or capillary. Occasionally, there are mixed types of vascular malformation. Also, they can be classified, according to the velocity of their flow, into high flow (arterial or arteriovenous) and low flow (venous, lymphatic, or capillary). The differentiation between these entities is critical for initiating treatment. Thus, hemangiomas are commonly responsive to systemic treatments, and vascular malformations are unresponsive. Moreover, the differentiation between high-flow and low-flow vascular malformations is also crucial to decide on adequate percutaneous embolization, or laser therapy that is commonly indicated in low-flow lesions.

On sonography, hemangiomas vary in their appearance according to the phase of the lesion. During the proliferative stage, they show as ill-defined, hypoechoic and/or heterogeneous and hypervascular lesions with arterial and venous flow and sometimes arteriovenous shunts. Occasionally, the peak systolic velocities in hemangiomas can be as high as in any other medium-size or large-size artery, such as the radial or external carotid arteries (**Fig. 12**). In the regression phase, the hemangiomas slowly turn to hyperechoic and hypovascular, appearing as a heterogeneous structure during the partial regression phase. Variable degrees of secondary atrophic or hypertrophic lipodystrophy (ie, abnormality in the content of fatty tissue) in the hypodermis may be detected in the total regression phase.[3,22–24]

Vascular malformations Vascular malformations commonly show as multichannel structures made up of anechoic, connecting vascular tract ducts (arterial or venous) or pseudocystic areas (venous or lymphatic), as hypoechoic areas in the dermis, or hyperechoic islands in the subcutaneous tissue (capillary). On color Doppler examination, the spectral curve analysis shows the characteristic arterial or venous flow patterns or the lack of flow in the lymphatic or capillary vascular malformations (**Figs. 13** and **14**). Mixed vascular malformations with more than one type of channel are also possible. Rarely, hyperechoic spots attributable to phleboliths are detected within the lesion. This is most commonly seen in venous vascular malformations. Importantly, sonography may provide information on the extension of the vascular lesion to deeper structures, such as glands, muscles, or cartilage, which may

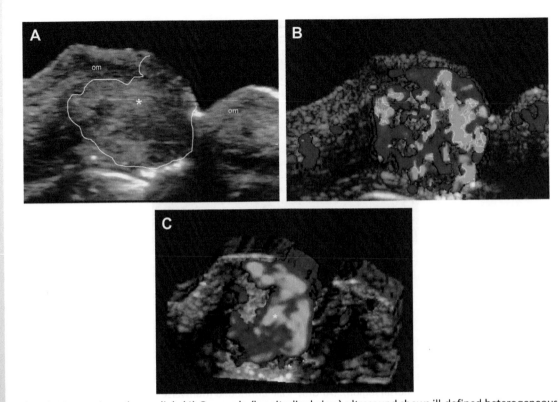

Fig. 12. Hemangioma (upper lip). (*A*) Gray-scale (longitudinal view) ultrasound shows ill-defined heterogeneous structure (*asterisk*) that affects the dermis and the orbicularis muscle (om). (*B*) Color Doppler ultrasound (longitudinal view) demonstrates strong hypervascularity within the lesion. (*C*) Three-dimensional power angio reconstruction highlights the lesional vessels (*asterisk*).

be critical in the vascular anomalies that present risky locations, such as the eyes, nose, or oral cavity. Additionally, ultrasound may be used to guide percutaneous procedures, such as embolization, and provide noninvasive data on the progress of systemic treatment. Hence, other imaging techniques, such as magnetic resonance imaging (MRI) can be reserved for the cases presenting multiple lesions and deep involvement.[3,25–27]

Malignant skin conditions

Nonmelanoma skin cancer Nonmelanoma skin cancer (NMSC), which includes both basal and squamous cell carcinoma, is the most common malignant tumor among human beings. Basal cell carcinoma (BCC) is the most frequent type and comprises 75% to 80% of the cases. Squamous cell carcinoma (SCC) is the second-most common type of skin cancer. Melanoma is the less frequent type but generates a high mortality rate and probably more medico-legal issues. Skin cancer is more common in areas of the body exposed to the sun and, therefore, can affect highly visible sites, such as the face, which can be of utmost importance in terms of the

cosmetic prognosis of the patient.[28] Moreover, incomplete excisions of primary NMSC lesions have been reported in up to 67% of the cases of SCC, and up to 32% in BCC.[29,30] Locations where the skin is thin, such as the eyelids, nose, ears, and lips can more easily involve deeper layers, for example muscle or cartilage. Hence, tumors measuring 2 cm or larger around the lips, ears, eyes, or nose have a poor prognosis.[28] Also, immunosuppressed patients under long-term treatment and/or those with chronic diseases, including the recipients of renal transplants, show a higher incidence of NMSC and this seems to be more aggressive.[31] Clinically, BCC appears as a slow-growing, painless, erythematous, pearly or ulcerated papule or nodule that can easily bleed. Additionally, BCC may present as a scarlike lesion. BCC rarely produce metastasis; however, it may generate local invasion. Clinically, SCC appears as a slow-growing, painless, erythematous, indurated, and readily bleeding lesion that can show a nodular, ulcerated, plaquelike, or verrucous surface. SCC is usually more aggressive on presentation compared with BCC and can show

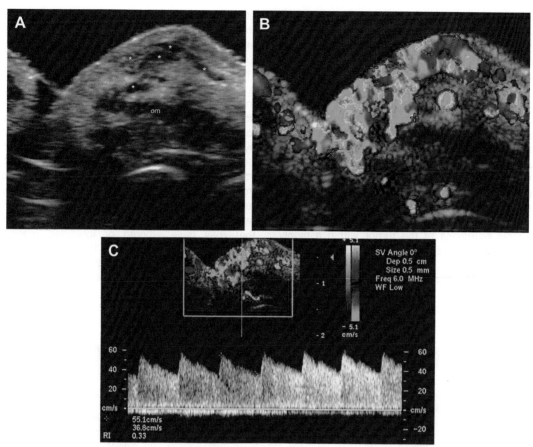

Fig. 13. High-flow arterial vascular malformation (lower lip). (*A*) Gray scale (longitudinal view) shows several anechoic ducts (*) that affect the dermis and the orbicularis muscle (om). (*B*) Color Doppler ultrasound (longitudinal view) demonstrates increased and turbulent blood flow within the lesional area. (*C*) Spectral curve analysis of the vessels (longitudinal view) shows arterial flow that presents a peak systolic velocity up to 55.1 cm/s.

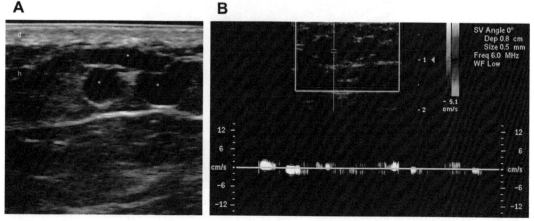

Fig. 14. Low-flow venous vascular malformation (posterior aspect of the right thigh). (*A*) Gray scale (transverse view) shows anechoic ducts and pseudocystic areas (*asterisks*) in the hypodermis. (*B*) Spectral curve analysis (transverse view) demonstrates low venous flow within the ducts. Abbreviations: d, dermis; h, hypodermis.

locoregional metastasis. On sonography, NMSC shows as a hypoechoic, heterogeneous lesion that may present irregular borders and, particularly in BCC lesions, some hyperechoic spots have been described. Thin, slow-flow arterial vessels are usually detected at the bottom of the lesion in BCC (**Fig. 15**); however, SCC can show more prominent vascularity within the lesion (**Fig. 16**). Two sonographic artifacts have been reported in BCC lesions. The first is produced by excessive surrounding inflammation that can generate a hypoechoic band with angles at the bottom of the lesion. The second artifact is usually seen in locations with hyperplastic sebaceous glands and may cause sonographic blurriness of the tumor within a highly heterogeneous tissue.[32,33]

Melanoma Melanoma comprises 4% to 11% of skin cancers but produces 75% of the deaths related to cutaneous malignant tumors.[34]

Moreover, recurrence has been described in the literature in up to 35.9% of the cases. An even higher rate of 46.1% may occur when the primary tumor is located in the head and neck region.[35] The most common form of clinical presentation is a dark hyperpigmented macule or nodule that may be associated with irregularities and ulceration. On sonography, melanoma appears as a fusiform hypoechoic lesion that frequently shows hypervascularity and locoregional invasion. Sonography can support the detection of satellite (<2 cm from the primary tumor), in transit (≥2 cm from the primary tumor), and nodal metastasis.[36–43] These secondary lesions can show as oval, hypoechoic, or heterogeneous structures that may have smooth or lobulated margins (**Fig. 17**).[44,45] Occasionally, these locoregional metastases may also show anechogenicity, and can mimic a collection of fluid or abscess. The latter appearance seems to be related to hypercellularity and not actual necrosis.[46]

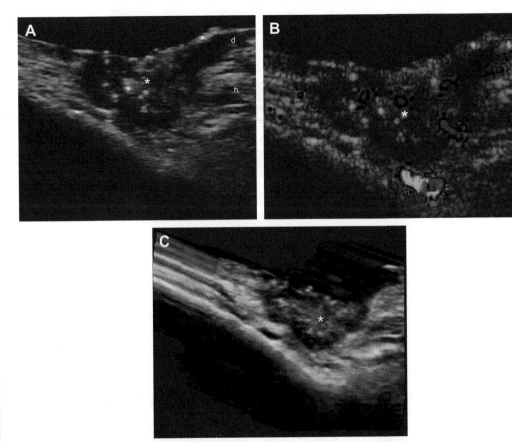

Fig. 15. Basal cell carcinoma (left paranasal region). (*A*) Gray-scale ultrasound (transverse view) shows hypoechoic lesion (*asterisk*) with irregular borders that involves epidermis, dermis, and upper hypodermis. Notice the hyperechoic spots within the tumor. (*B*) Color Doppler ultrasound (transverse axis) demonstrates slightly increased vascularity within the lesion with thin vessels. (*C*) Three-dimensional reconstruction (5–8 seconds sweep, transverse axis) of the tumor (*asterisk*).

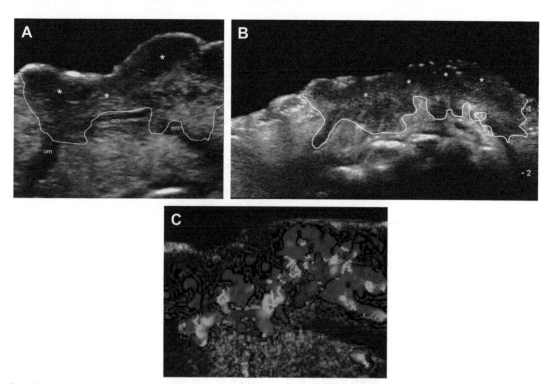

Fig. 16. Squamous cell carcinoma (lower lip). (*A*) Gray-scale ultrasound shows ill-defined and irregular hypoe-choic structure (*asterisks*) that affects the dermis and orbicularis muscle (om). (*B*) Gray-scale ultrasound, showing an extended and outlined transverse view of the tumor (*asterisks*). (*C*) Color Doppler ultrasound demonstrates strong vascularity within the lesion.

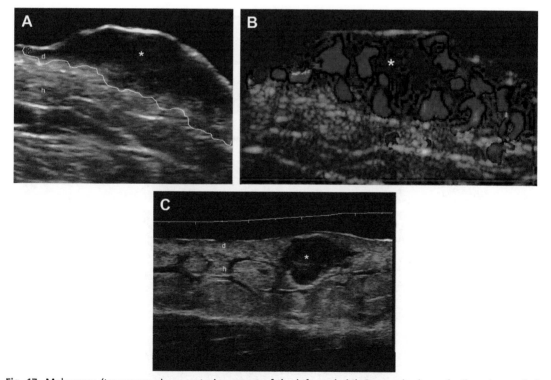

Fig. 17. Melanoma (transverse view, posterior aspect of the left arm). (*A*) Gray scale shows fusiform hypoechoic lesion (*asterisk*, outlined) that involves dermis and part of the upper hypodermis. (*B*) Color Doppler ultrasound demonstrates prominent vascularity within the tumor (*asterisk*). (*C*) Gray scale (longitudinal view) demonstrates a hypoechoic dermal and hypodermal nodule (*asterisk*) with lobulated and slightly irregular borders that corre-sponds to an in-transit metastasis (≥2 cm from the primary tumor). Anechoic bands with fluid suggestive of inter-lobular edema in the hypodermis are also detected.

Thus, the assessment of the depth of the primary cutaneous melanoma may affect important presurgical decisions, such as the size of the incision, or the performance of a sentinel node procedure (indicated in melanomas deeper than 1 mm). Moreover, the presence of secondary lesions seems to be more related to the biologic characteristics of the primary tumor rather than the size of the surgical excision.[47]

Inflammatory Conditions

Plantar warts

Plantar warts are infectious conditions caused by the human papilloma virus (HPV) and clinically appear as hyperkeratotic lesions in the sole of the foot. Plantar warts can be extremely painful; therefore, may clinically simulate other conditions, such as foreign bodies or Morton neuromas.

On sonography, the classical appearance is a fusiform hypoechoic lesion located in the epidermis and dermis. Variable degrees of hypervascularity may be detected at the bottom of these lesions and a concomitant secondary plantar bursitis may also be found underneath the wart (**Fig. 18**).[48,49]

Foreign Bodies

Foreign bodies are exogenous components that can be classified according to their composition into organic (ie, derived from living organisms, such as splinters of wood or rose thorns) or inert (eg, pieces of glass or metal). Foreign bodies are commonly introduced during a traumatic event that occasionally may not be noticed or spontaneously mentioned by the patient, especially when this condition affects children or babies. Clinically, foreign bodies may show as painless or painful, erythematous or skin-colored bumps. On sonography, foreign bodies commonly appear as a bilaminar or laminar hyperechoic band that in the case of inert materials can present a posterior reverberance artifact. Hypoechoic inflamed and granulomatous tissue usually surrounds the exogenous component. On color Doppler examination, slow-flow vessels can be detected on the periphery of the foreign deposit (**Fig. 19**). Sonography can confirm the diagnosis, assess the nature of the exogenous material and its exact location, and finally guide its percutaneous removal.[3,50,51]

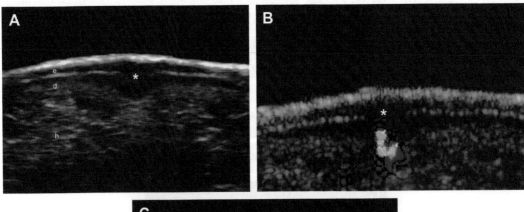

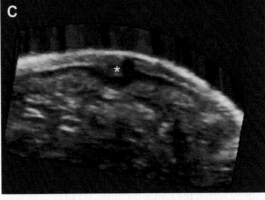

Fig. 18. Plantar wart (left foot). (*A*) Gray scale shows hypoechoic fusiform lesion that affects epidermis and dermis (*asterisk*). (*B*) Color Doppler ultrasound demonstrates increased blood flow within the lesion. (*C*) Three-dimensional reconstruction (5–8 seconds sweep) of the lesion. e, epidermis; d, dermis; h, hypodermis.

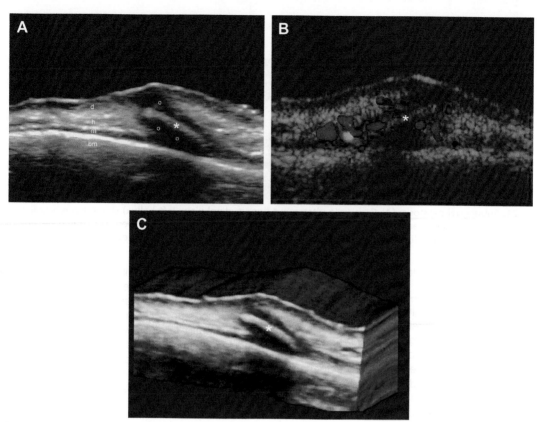

Fig. 19. Foreign body (splinter of wood, frontal region). (*A*) Gray scale ultrasound (transverse view) demonstrates hyperechoic band that corresponds to a foreign body (*) surrounded by hypoechoic granulomatous tissue (o). (*B*) Color Doppler ultrasound (oblique view) shows increased vascularity in the periphery of the foreign body (*). (*C*) Three-dimensional reconstruction (5–8 seconds sweep, transverse view) of the lesional area (*). bm, bony margin of the skull; d, dermis; e, epidermis; h, hypodermis; m, epicranious muscle.

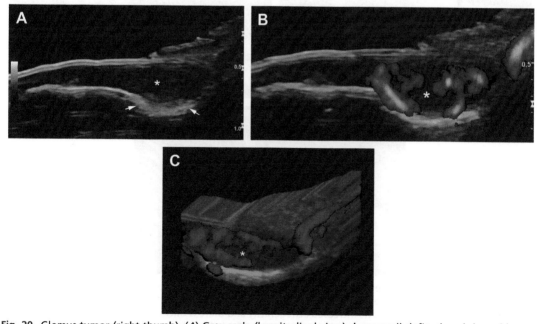

Fig. 20. Glomus tumor (right thumb). (*A*) Gray scale (longitudinal view) shows well defined oval-shaped hypoechoic nodule (*asterisk*) that affects the proximal nail bed and produces scalloping of the bony margin of the distal phalanx (*arrows*). (*B*) Power Doppler ultrasound (longitudinal view) demonstrates increased blood flow within the nodule. (*C*) Three-dimensional power angio reconstruction of the tumor (5–8 seconds sweep).

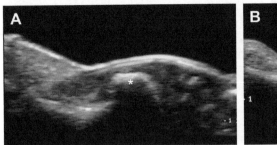
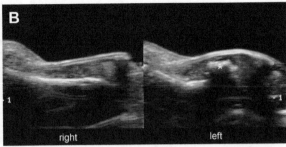

Fig. 21. Subungual exostosis. (*A*) Gray-scale ultrasound (longitudinal view, left hallux) shows hyperechoic band (*asterisk*) with posterior acoustic shadowing artifact that protrudes into the nail bed. (*B*) Gray-scale side-by-side comparison (longitudinal view) clearly demonstrates the lesion (*asterisk*) in the left subungual region.

UNGUAL AND PERIUNGUAL CONDITIONS
Glomus Tumor

Glomus tumors are benign entities derived from the neuromyoarterial apparatus and commonly affect the nail bed. Clinically, glomus tumors frequently present as an extremely painful nail with hypersensitivity to cold. Sometimes secondary deformation of the nail plate can be detected.[52] Recurrence in patients without presurgical imaging has been reported in up to 20% of the cases. A high correlation between ultrasound and intraoperative size of the tumors has been described in the literature, which includes submillimeter lesions.[53]

On sonography, glomus tumor usually appears as a centrally located, well-defined, hypoechoic nodule in the nail bed with scalloping of the bony margin of the distal phalanx. The proximal nail bed is more commonly affected than the distal region. On color Doppler examination, it frequently shows hypervascularity (**Fig. 20**). Nevertheless,

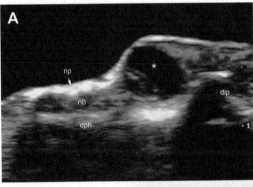
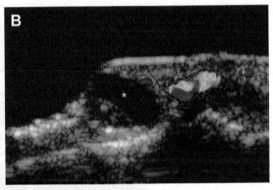
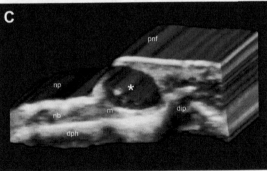

Fig. 22. Synovial cyst (left middle finger). (*A*) Gray scale (longitudinal view) shows well-defined, oval-shaped, anechoic structure (*asterisk*) in the proximal nail fold. The cyst (*asterisk*) presents echoes (debris) and compresses the matrix region. The nail bed shows increased echogenicity and there is thickening of the nail plate with loss of the bilaminar pattern. (*B*) Color Doppler ultrasound (longitudinal view) demonstrates lack of vascularity within the cyst (*). (*C*) Three-dimensional reconstruction (5–8 seconds sweep) that highlights the cyst (*) and the secondary changes in the nail unit. *Abbreviations:* dip, distal interphalangeal joint; dph, distal phalanx; m, ungual matrix; nb, nail bed; np, nail plates; pnf, proximal nail fold.

there are some rare variants that can show hypovascularity.[6,53–56]

Subungual Exostosis

Subungual exostosis is an overgrowth of bone arising from the distal phalanx and protruding into the nail bed. Occasionally, the bony structure can be accompanied by a cartilaginous cap (osteochondroma). Clinically, subungual exostosis commonly shows as a painless or painful erythematous subungual lump, sometimes with dystrophy of the nail plates.[57] Nevertheless, clinically, subungual exostosis can be a potent simulator of other common ungual conditions, such as glomus tumor or onychomycosis. This characteristic may be the reason why these cases are frequently first referred for ultrasound examination rather than directly for x-rays.

On sonography, they show as a hyperechoic line or band connected to the bony margin of the distal phalanx that commonly displaces the nail plates upward and produces posterior acoustic shadowing. If cartilage is associated with the bone, a hypoechoic cap can be detected in the surface of this bandlike structure. Frequently, there is thickening and hypoechogenicity of the nail bed, secondary to the inflammation and granulomatous reaction. These exostoses may also extend to the periungual tissue and generate hypoechogenicity of the dermis. On color Doppler examination, the nail bed is usually hypovascular (**Fig. 21**).[6,58]

Synovial Cyst

Also called myxoid cysts, synovial cysts are fluid-filled structures commonly associated with osteoarthrosis and/or synovitis of the distal interphalangeal joint (DIP). Thus, the leakage of fluid and/or synovial proliferation toward the ungual region can clinically produce a periungual erythematous, firm swelling or lump.[59] Concavity and/or dystrophy of the nail plate in the same axis as the cyst are commonly seen, secondary to compression of the ungual matrix by this cystic structure. Occasionally, these synovial cysts can protrude into the nail bed. On sonography, they show as a round or oval-shaped, well-defined, anechoic structure connected through a thin, usually serpiginous tract to the DIP. Posterior acoustic transmission is frequently detected and on color Doppler examination, there is a lack of flow within the cyst[6,58] (**Fig. 22**).

SUMMARY

Ultrasound provides relevant anatomic data in common cutaneous and ungual lesions. This information may support the medical or surgical treatment and improve the cosmetic result of the patient.

REFERENCES

1. Wortsman X, Wortsman J. Clinical usefulness of variable-frequency ultrasound in localized lesions of the skin. J Am Acad Dermatol 2010;62:247–56.
2. Farinelli N, Berardesca E. The skin integument: variation relative to sex, race, and body region. In: Serup J, Jemec GB, Grove GL, editors. Handbook of noninvasive methods and the skin. Boca Raton (FL): Taylor and Francis; 2006. p. 27–36.
3. Wortsman X. Common applications of dermatologic sonography. J Ultrasound Med 2012;31:97–111.
4. Mc Gonagle D, Tan AL, Benjamin M. The nail as musculoskeletal appendage—implications for an improved understanding of the link between psoriasis and arthritis. Dermatology 2009;218:97–102.
5. Wortsman X, Jemec GB. Ultrasound imaging of nails. Dermatol Clin 2006;24:323–8.
6. Wortsman X, Wortsman J, Soto R, et al. Benign tumors and pseudotumors of the nail: a novel application of sonography. J Ultrasound Med 2010;29:803–16.
7. Wortsman X, Wortsman J, Matsuoka L, et al. Sonography in pathologies of scalp and hair. Br J Radiol 2012;85:647–55.
8. Jin W, Ryu KN, Kim GY, et al. Sonographic findings of ruptured epidermal inclusion cysts in superficial soft tissue: emphasis on shapes, pericystic changes, and pericystic vascularity. J Ultrasound Med 2008;27:171–6.
9. Huang CC, Ko SF, Huang HY, et al. Epidermal cysts in the superficial soft tissue: sonographic features with an emphasis on the pseudotestis pattern. J Ultrasound Med 2011;30:11–7.
10. Folpe AL, Reisenauer AK, Mentzel T, et al. Proliferating trichilemmal tumors: clinicopathologic evaluation is a guide to biologic behavior. J Cutan Pathol 2003;30:492–8.
11. Mentes O, Oysul A, Harlak A, et al. Ultrasonography accurately evaluates the dimension and shape of the pilonidal sinus. Clinics (Sao Paulo) 2009;64:189–92.
12. Fornage BD, Tassin GB. Sonographic appearances of superficial soft tissue lipomas. J Clin Ultrasound 1991;19:215–20.
13. Kuwano Y, Ishizaki K, Watanabe R, et al. Efficacy of diagnostic ultrasonography of lipomas, epidermal cysts, and ganglions. Arch Dermatol 2009;145:761–4.
14. Lee JY, Kim SM, Fessell DP, et al. Sonography of benign palpable masses of the elbow. J Ultrasound Med 2011;30:1113–9.
15. Roche NA, Monstrey SJ, Matton GE. Pilomatricoma in children: common but often misdiagnosed. Acta Chir Belg 2010;110:250–4.

16. Hwang JY, Lee SW, Lee SM. The common ultrasonographic features of pilomatricoma. J Ultrasound Med 2005;24:1397–402.

17. Choo HJ, Lee SJ, Lee YH, et al. Pilomatricomas: the diagnostic value of ultrasound. Skeletal Radiol 2010;39:243–50.

18. Solivetti FM, Elia F, Drusco A, et al. Epithelioma of Malherbe: new ultrasound patterns. J Exp Clin Cancer Res 2010;29:42.

19. Wortsman X, Wortsman J, Arellano J, et al. Pilomatrixomas presenting as vascular tumors on color Doppler ultrasound. J Pediatr Surg 2010;45:2094–8.

20. MacKee P, Calonje E, Granter S. Tumors of fibrous and myofibroblastic tissue. In: MacKee P, Calonje E, Granter S, editors. Pathology of the skin with clinical correlation. 3rd edition. Elsevier Mosby; 2005. p. 1669–723.

21. Mulliken JB, Glowacki J. Hemangiomas and vascular malformations in infants and children: a classification based on endothelial characteristics. Plast Reconstr Surg 1982;69:412–22.

22. Enjolras O. Classification and management of the various superficial vascular anomalies: hemangiomas and vascular malformations. J Dermatol 1997;24:701–10.

23. Dubois J, Patriquin HB, Garel L, et al. Soft tissue hemangiomas in infants and children: diagnosis using Doppler sonography. Am J Roentgenol 1998;171:247–52.

24. Paltiel HJ, Burrows PE, Kozakewich HP, et al. Soft tissue vascular anomalies: utility of US for diagnosis. Radiology 2000;214:747–54.

25. Puig S, Casati B, Staudenherz A, et al. Vascular low-flow malformations in children: current concepts for classification, diagnosis and therapy. Eur J Radiol 2005;53:35–45.

26. Trop I, Dubois J, Guibaud L, et al. Soft tissue venous malformations in pediatric and young adult patients: diagnosis with Doppler US. Radiology 1999;212:841–5.

27. Dubois J, Soulez G, Oliva VL, et al. Soft-tissue venous malformations in adult patients: imaging and therapeutic issues. Radiographics 2001;21:1519–31.

28. Gniadecki R, Normal Dam T. Basal cell carcinoma—clinical guidelines, Danish Dermatological Society. Forum Nordic Derm Venereol 2009;14:4–6.

29. Matteucci P, Pinder R, Magdum A, et al. Accuracy in skin lesion diagnosis and the exclusion of malignancy. J Plast Reconstr Aesthet Surg 2011;64:1460–5.

30. Santiago F, Serra D, Vieira R, et al. Incidence and factors associated with recurrence after incomplete excision of basal cell carcinomas: a study of 90 cases. J Eur Acad Dermatol Venereol 2010;24:1421–4.

31. Zavos G, Karidis NP, Tsourouflis G, et al. Nonmelanoma skin cancer after renal transplantation: a single-center experience in 1736 transplantations. Int J Dermatol 2011;50:1496–500.

32. Bobadilla F, Wortsman X, Muñoz C, et al. Pre-surgical high resolution ultrasound of facial basal cell carcinoma: correlation with histology. Cancer Imaging 2008;8:163–72.

33. Uhara H, Hayashi K, Koga H, et al. Multiple hypersonographic spots in basal cell carcinoma. Dermatol Surg 2007;33:1215–9.

34. Reintgen DS, Vollmer R, Tso CY, et al. Prognosis for recurrent stage I malignant melanoma. Arch Surg 1987;122:1338–42.

35. Nazarian LN, Alexander AA, Kurtz AB, et al. Superficial melanoma metastases: appearances on gray-scale and color Doppler sonography. AJR Am J Roentgenol 1998;170:459–63.

36. Wortsman X. Sonography of the primary cutaneous melanoma: a review. Radiol Res Pract 2012;2012:814396.

37. Tacke J, Haagen G, Horstein O, et al. Clinical relevance of sonometry-derived tumour thickness in malignant melanoma—a statistical analysis. Br J Dermatol 1995;132:209–14.

38. Kaikaris V, Samsanavičius D, Kęstutis M, et al. Measurement of melanoma thickness—comparison of two methods: ultrasound versus morphology. J Plast Reconstr Aesthet Surg 2011;64:796–802.

39. Catalano O, Siani A. Cutaneous melanoma: role of ultrasound in the assessment of locoregional spread. Curr Probl Diagn Radiol 2010;39:30–6.

40. Vilana R, Puig S, Sanchez M, et al. Preoperative assessment of cutaneous melanoma thickness using 10-MHz sonography. AJR Am J Roentgenol 2009;193:639–43.

41. Music MM, Hertl K, Kadivec M, et al. Pre-operative ultrasound with a 12-15 MHz linear probe reliably differentiates between melanoma thicker and thinner than 1 mm. J Eur Acad Dermatol Venereol 2010;24:1105–8.

42. Lassau N, Mercier S, Koscielny S, et al. Prognostic value of high-frequency sonography and color Doppler sonography for the preoperative assessment of melanomas. AJR Am J Roentgenol 1999;172:457–61.

43. Lassau N, Koscielny S, Avril MF, et al. Prognostic value of angiogenesis evaluated with high-frequency and color Doppler sonography for preoperative assessment of melanomas. AJR Am J Roentgenol 2002;178:1547–51.

44. Voit C, Van Akkooi AC, Schäfer-Hesterberg G, et al. Ultrasound morphology criteria predict metastatic disease of the sentinel nodes in patients with melanoma. J Clin Oncol 2010;28:847–52.

45. Nazarian L, Alexander AA, Rawool NM, et al. Malignant melanoma: impact of superficial US on management. Radiology 1996;199:273–7.

46. Catalano O, Voit C, Sandomenico F, et al. Previously reported sonographic appearances of regional melanoma metastases are not likely due to necrosis. J Ultrasound Med 2011;30:1041–9.

47. Clemente-Ruiz de Almiron A, Serrano-Ortega S. Risk factors for in-transit metastasis in patients with cutaneous melanoma. Actas Dermosifiliogr 2012;103: 207–13 [in Spanish].

48. Wortsman X, Jemec GB, Sazunic I. Anatomical detection of inflammatory changes associated with plantar warts by ultrasound. Dermatology 2010; 220:213–7.

49. Wortsman X, Sazunic I, Jemec GB. Sonography of plantar warts: role in diagnosis and treatment. J Ultrasound Med 2009;28:787–93.

50. Halaas GW. Management of foreign bodies in the skin. Am Fam Physician 2007;76:683–8.

51. Valle M, Zamorani MP. Skin and subcutaneous tissue. In: Bianchi S, Martinoli C, editors. Ultrasound of the musculoskeletal system. Berlin: Springer-Verlag; 2007. p. 27–31.

52. Baran R, Haneke E, Drape JL, et al. Tumors of the nail and adjacent tissues. In: Baran R, Dawber RP, de Berker D, et al, editors. Diseases of the nails and their management. 3rd edition. Oxford: Blackwell and Science; 2001. p. 515–601.

53. Wortsman X, Jemec GB. Role of high-variable frequency ultrasound in preoperative diagnosis of glomus tumors: a pilot study. Am J Clin Dermatol 2009;10:23–7.

54. Chen SH, Chen YL, Cheng MH, et al. The use of ultrasonography in preoperative localization of digital glomus tumors. Plast Reconstr Surg 2003; 112:115–9.

55. Matsunaga A, Ochiai T, Abe I, et al. Subungual glomus tumour: evaluation of ultrasound imaging in preoperative assessment. Eur J Dermatol 2007;17: 67–9.

56. Baek HJ, Lee SJ, Cho KH, et al. Subungual tumors: clinicopathologic correlation with US and MR imaging findings. Radiographics 2010;30:1621–36.

57. García Carmona FJ, Pascual Huerta J, Fernández Morato D. A proposed subungual exostosis clinical classification and treatment plan. J Am Podiatr Med Assoc 2009;99:519–24.

58. Wortsman X, Wortsman J. Skin ultrasound, chapter 9. In: Dogra V, Gaitini D, editors. Musculoskeletal ultrasound with CT and MRI correlation. 1st edition. Thieme; 2010. p. 147–70.

59. Kuflik EG. Specific indications for cryosurgery of the nail unit. Myxoid cysts and periungual verrucae. J Dermatol Surg Oncol 1992;18:702–6.

Rheumatologic Applications of Musculoskeletal Ultrasonography

Ralf G. Thiele, MD

KEYWORDS

- Ultrasound • Ultrasonography • Sonography • Synovitis • Rheumatoid arthritis • Gout • Enthesitis
- Erosions

KEY POINTS

- Ultrasonography is an imaging modality that identifies both bony contour and soft tissues.
- Proliferative synovial tissue should be examined both with gray-scale and color/power Doppler ultrasonography.
- Ultrasonography distinguishes mechanical enthesopathy from spondyloarthritis-associated enthesitis.
- Monosodium urate tophi and calcium-containing crystal aggregates can be identified sonographically.
- Ultrasonography is used in the follow-up of synovial proliferation and hyperemia to monitor treatment response.
- Standardization of the examination is achieved through adherence to guidelines.
- Training is offered by the European League Against Rheumatism, the Ultrasound School of North American Rheumatologists, and the American College of Rheumatology (ACR).
- Certification of individuals is offered by the American Registry for Diagnostic Medical Sonography or the ACR.
- Accreditation of practices is granted by the American Institute of Ultrasound in Medicine.

INTRODUCTION

Musculoskeletal (MSK) ultrasonography has become a premier imaging modality in rheumatology over the last 20 years.[1] Rheumatologists are one of the largest groups of users of MSK ultrasonography. Much of the literature on MSK ultrasonography has investigated rheumatologic indications (**Fig. 1**). Among the different imaging modalities, MSK ultrasonography receives the greatest attention of rheumatology researchers (**Fig. 2**). Trained examiners reach good to very good agreement when obtaining and evaluating ultrasound images.[2–4] In a large cohort study comparing agreement of interpretation of ultrasonography, magnetic resonance (MR) imaging, and computed

tomography (CT), ultrasonography had significantly lower rates of discrepancy than MR imaging and CT (**Box 1**).[5] When ultrasonography is performed to assess synovitis using gray-scale or power ultrasound, there also appears to be less intraobserver variability (the same examiner evaluating a standard set of joints twice with a 2–4-day interval) with ultrasonography when compared with a standardized clinical examination of the same joints (**Table 1**).[6]

High-frequency ultrasonography (using transducer frequencies of 12–18 MHz) is particularly well suited to detect abnormality in rheumatic conditions. Superficially located soft-tissue structures can be seen in greater detail than by MR imaging (spatial resolution 0.15 mm at 10 MHz vs

Department of Medicine, Allergy/Immunology & Rheumatology Division, University of Rochester School of Medicine and Dentistry, 601 Elmwood Avenue, Box 695, Rochester, NY 14642, USA
E-mail address: ralf_thiele@urmc.rochester.edu

Ultrasound Clin 7 (2012) 525–535
http://dx.doi.org/10.1016/j.cult.2012.08.008
1556-858X/12/$ – see front matter © 2012 Elsevier Inc. All rights reserved.

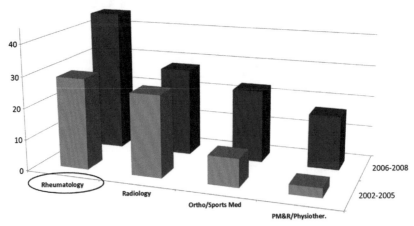

Fig. 1. Publications on musculoskeletal ultrasonography. Affiliation of first author. Listings in OVID with search terms "musculoskeletal" AND "ultrasound."

0.45 mm). Conventional radiography, still the mainstay of imaging in rheumatology, is used to detect typical erosions or new bone formation, but soft-tissue structures are poorly visualized. Nevertheless, even the main indication for conventional radiography in rheumatic diseases, detection of erosions in rheumatoid arthritis, is less successful when compared with ultrasonography. Particularly in early disease, when therapeutic decisions are critical in helping prevent future joint damage, ultrasonography detects 6.5 times the number of erosions when compared with conventional radiography, in 7.5-fold the number of patients.[7]

INDICATIONS

Typical indications for the use of MSK ultrasonography in rheumatology include:

- Assessment of synovitis and tenosynovitis
- Detection of bony erosions
- Soft-tissue rheumatism
- Crystal arthritis[8]

- Enthesitis in spondyloarthropathies[9,10]
- Disease monitoring
- Assessment of treatment response
- Procedure guidance in ultrasonography for diagnostic and therapeutic purposes[11,12]

Less common indications for ultrasonography in rheumatology are:

- Diagnosis of large-vessel vasculitis including giant-cell arteritis (temporal arteritis) and Takayasu arteritis[13,14]
- Assessment of vascularization in Raynaud phenomenon[15]
- Assessment of skin thickness and tendon friction rubs in scleroderma
- Distinction of fibromyalgia (negative examination) and inflammatory arthritis

---

Box 1
Interpretation of ultrasonography: better agreement than MR imaging and CT

- 21,482 consecutive CT, MR, and ultrasonography studies
- Read by on-call fourth-year radiology resident
- Read by subspecialty radiologist
- MR and CT interpretations had significantly higher rates of discrepancy than ultrasonography
- Discrepancy rates:
  - MR, 1.4%; CT, 0.9%; ultrasonography, 0.2%; $P<.001$

Data from Ruma J, Klein KA, Chong S, et al. Cross-sectional examination interpretation discrepancies between oncall diagnostic radiology residents and subspecialty faculty radiologists: analysis by imaging modality and subspecialty. J Am Coll Radiol 2011;8(6):409–14.

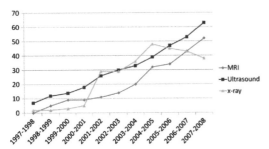

Fig. 2. Publications in rheumatology using imaging. OVID search stratified by years: MRI AND Rheumatology; (Ultrasound OR Ultrasonography OR Sonography) AND Rheumatology; (Radiography OR x-ray) AND Rheumatology.

Table 1
Intraobserver reliability of ultrasonographic scoring systems

Scoring System	ICC (95% CI)	Weighted κ (95% CI)
20-joint count: clinical examination	0.60 (−008 to 0.90)	0.56 (−0.07–1.00)
20 joints ultrasound B-mode	0.85 (0.45–0.97)	0.83 (0.62–1.00)
20 joints ultrasound power Doppler	0.96 (0.83–0.99)	0.95 (0.91–1.00)

Intraobserver reliability of the different clinical and ultrasonographic scoring systems was evaluated twice with a 2- to 4-day interval in patients with rheumatoid arthritis. Reliability is at least as good as for clinical measures.
Abbreviations: CI, confidence interval; ICC, intraclass correlation coefficient.
Data from Dougados M, Jousse-Joulin S, Mistretta F, et al. Evaluation of several ultrasonography scoring systems for synovitis and comparison to clinical examination: results from a prospective multicentre study of rheumatoid arthritis. Ann Rheum Dis 2010;69(5):828–33.

- Assessment of major salivary glands in Sjögren syndrome[16]
- Others

ANATOMY
Synovial Joints

The following anatomic structures are relevant for the sonographic assessment of joints (**Figs. 3** and **4**):

- Bony contour. This structure has a hyperechoic appearance. The histologically rough, textured bone surface reflects sound waves in different directions. No anisotropy is seen if bony surfaces are insonated from different angles.
- Hyaline cartilage. The high water content leads to an anechoic to hypoechoic appearance (depending on gain settings). Hyaline cartilage covers the bony surfaces in synovial joints.
- Synovial lining. The synovial lining of the fibrous joint capsule is only 1 to 3 cell layers strong and is not typically seen sonographically. Finding of hypoechoic synovial tissue is abnormal in healthy controls.
- Joint capsule. The fibrous joint capsule has a hyperechoic appearance. Typically there is a proximal reserve fold, or duplication of the capsule to allow flexion and extension.

The distal end of the joint capsule is generally firmly attached at the base of the distal bone.
- Overlying tendon. In finger joints, which are often affected by rheumatoid arthritis, flexor and extensor tendons cover the joint capsule in close proximity. Tenosynovitis can affect the flexor tendons of the fingers. The dorsal extensor tendons are devoid of a tendon sheath and can therefore, by definition, not be affected by tenosynovitis. Paratenonitis can be observed once synovial tissue breaks through the dorsal capsule.

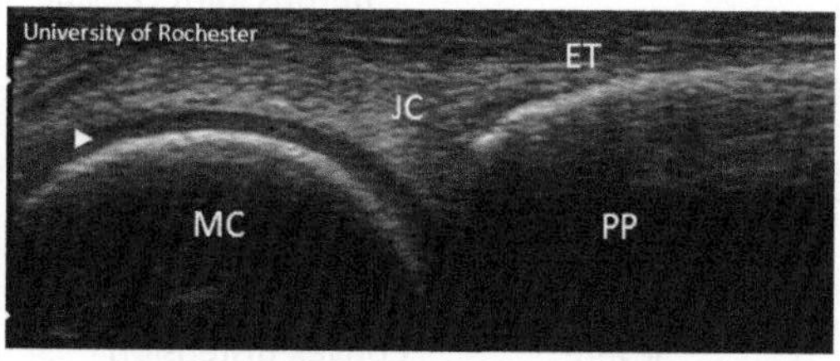

Tenosynovium

Where tendons cross joint areas with substantial range of motion, particularly wrists and ankles, they are supplied with a protective sheath. Tendon and sheath share anatomic characteristics with synovial joints, and are as commonly affected by inflammatory arthritis.

- The fibrous tendon sheath has an inner lining of synovial tissue, and the tendon itself is lined with a layer of synovial tissue.

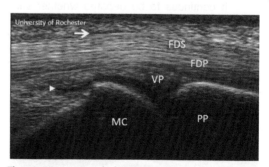

Fig. 4. Metacarpophalangeal joint. Volar long-axis view. Healthy control. Arrow points to A1 pulley. Arrowhead points to proximal volar recess of joint. FDP, flexor digitorum profundus tendon; FDS, flexor digitorum superficialis tendon; MC, metacarpal head; PP, proximal phalanx; VP, volar plate.

Fig. 3. Metacarpophalangeal joint. Dorsal long-axis view. Healthy control. Arrowhead indicates hyaline cartilage. ET, extensor tendon; JC, joint capsule; MC, metacarpal head; PP, proximal phalanx.

- Both synovial layers are connected by the mesotendineum.
- Blood supply to synovial tissue and tendon runs through this synovial duplication.
- The interspace between inner and outer synovial layers may fill with synovial fluid or proliferative synovial tissue.

Enthesis Organ

At tendon attachment points, different tissues help provide protection to adjacent bone and allow proper functioning (**Fig. 5**). As these tissues function in concert, the term enthesis organ has been coined.[17,18]

- Tendons frequently insert at an acute angle into bones. Therefore, the most distal portion of the fibers has to curve down to meet the bone. This change of direction of reflection can lead to profound anisotropy near tendon attachments, as in the Achilles tendon. Adjustment of transducer position (head-heel tilt) can overcome this artifact.
- Portions of cortical cortex can be covered with cartilage, to help deflect shear stress of tendon on bone. This cartilage is most pronounced over the calcaneus, near the Achilles tendon insertion, the area of greatest mechanical stress.
- The retrocalcaneal bursa fills out the triangular space between Achilles tendon insertion and periosteal fibrocartilage. Bursal fat can slide in and out of this triangular space, with range of motion of the ankle, to further help cushioning against mechanical impact. The bursal capsule is lined with synovial tissue that may produce increased fluid or proliferate in inflammatory arthritis.
- Bony erosions at the calcaneus are often seen more readily using ultrasonography in comparison with conventional radiography. It continues to be debated whether such erosions outside of synovial joints in spondyloarthropathies are caused by a primary bone marrow lesion, or if they are rather caused by invading synovial tissue from adjacent synovial structures such as bursae.

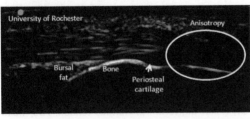

Fig. 5. Insertion of Achilles tendon. Dorsal long-axis view. Healthy control.

IMAGING PROTOCOLS

1. For the sonographic screening for rheumatoid arthritis, the following protocol allows for a high yield of detecting tenosynovitis and synovitis:

   a. Determine the clinically more affected hand (more joints or tendons sheaths with redness, swelling, or warmth and tenderness on range of motion)

   b. Assess for tenosynovitis in dorsal long-axis midline view (over extensor compartment 4) and ulnar long-axis view (over extensor carpi ulnaris tendon)

   c. Assess for synovitis in dorsal long-axis views over metacarpophalangeal (MCP) joints 2–5

   d. Assess for synovitis in volar long-axis views in proximal interphalangeal (PIP) joints 2–5

   e. Identify distention of joint capsule or tendon sheath in gray scale first, then assess abnormal tissue for hyperemia using color or power Doppler ultrasonography

   f. Findings can be documented as present or absent, or semiquantitatively using a scale ranging from 0 to 3

2. A different screening protocol uses assessment of 7 joints (US7)[19]:

The US7 score includes the clinically dominant wrist, MCP and PIP joints 2 and 3, metatarsophalangeal (MTP) joint 2, and 5 joints that are evaluated for synovitis, tenosynovitis/paratenonitis, and erosions from the dorsal and palmar/plantar aspects by gray-scale and power Doppler ultrasonography. Additional lateral scans are performed at MCP 2 and MTP 5.

Grading of Synovitis

Grade		
0	No gray-scale change	
1	Mild synovitis	Small anechoic or hyperechoic line beneath hyperechoic fibrous joint capsule
2	Moderate synovitis	Joint capsule is distended. Remains parallel to bony contour up to straightening out of the convexity of joint recesses
3	Severe synovitis	Convex distension of joint capsule

DIAGNOSTIC CRITERIA

Tables 2–6.

Table 2
Synovitis

	Definition	Sonographic Appearance	Examples of Rheumatic Diseases
Synovial effusion	Distension of interval between hyperechoic bony contour and hyperechoic, fibrous joint capsule by synovial fluid	Anechoic (occasionally hypoechoic if high cell count), displaceable with transducer pressure	Inflammatory arthritis including RA or PsA, early stages. Noninflammatory arthritis including osteoarthritis
Synovial proliferation	Thickening of synovial lining tissue emanating from hyperechoic fibrous joint capsule	Hypoechoic, villous, or diffuse proliferative. Slightly compressible with transducer pressure but not displaceable	Particularly inflammatory arthritis including RA and PsA. Not typical for gout. Occasionally seen in OA, particularly in knee
Synovial hyperemia	Pulse synchronous Doppler signal that is seen over area identified as synovial tissue on gray-scale ultrasonography		Inflammatory arthritis including RA and PsA. Rarely OA. Doppler signals can also be seen adjacent to gouty tophi

Abbreviations: OA, osteoarthritis; PsA, psoriatic arthritis; RA, rheumatoid arthritis.

Table 3
Soft-tissue rheumatism

	Definition	Sonographic Appearance	Examples of Rheumatic Diseases
Bursitis	Physiologic or adventitial synovial sac between tendon, ligament, muscle and bone	Anechoic fluid collection in typical anatomic location. Fluid may be displaceable with transducer pressure	Polymyalgia rheumatica: bursitis in hip and shoulder girdle. Olecranon and prepatellar bursitis in gout
Mechanical enthesopathy	Thickening of tendon above physiologic measures[35]	Loss of densely packed fibrillar pattern. May find irregular bony contour at attachment point. Small calcium deposits in tendon body near attachment. Doppler studies may show hyperemia, typically not at interface of tendon and bone	Lateral epicondylitis, jumper's knee, Achilles tendinosis, plantar fasciitis
Fibromyalgia	Widespread musculoskeletal pain associated with typical tender points and nonrestorative sleep, negative serology	Absence of synovial effusion, thickening and hyperemia. Sonographic findings same as healthy controls	Distinguish chronic pain syndromes from inflammatory arthritis

Table 4
Crystal arthritis

	Description	Sonographic Appearance	Rheumatic Condition
Monosodium urate tophi	Aggregates of monosodium urate crystals in or around joints, tendons, and bursae	Usually hyperechoic, slightly inhomogeneous, often oval-shaped bodies with anechoic rim	Gout
Double contour sign	Layer of monosodium urate crystals over hyaline cartilage	Hyperechoic layer covering the anechoic or hypoechoic hyaline cartilage over hyperechoic bony contour	Gout
Chondrocalcinosis	Calcium pyrophosphate deposition in central lacunes of hyaline cartilage or fibrocartilage	Hyperechoic aggregates of crystals layering in the center of anechoic hyaline cartilage or hyperechoic fibrocartilage	Pseudogout

PATHOLOGY

Erosions

Historically, detection of typical erosions on conventional radiography was a main criterion for the diagnosis of rheumatoid arthritis, gout, spondyloarthritis, and other arthropathies (**Figs. 6** and **7**). Because conventional radiography projects 3-dimensional structures on 2-dimensional films, bony erosions need to be seen in profile to be accurately characterized. Sonography, as a cross-sectional and dynamic imaging modality (the transducer can be led partially around bony structures such as metacarpal heads), detects more erosions in rheumatoid arthritis and gout than does conventional radiography.[7,23] As ultrasonography also detects as>sociated tissues that are involved in erosion formation, detection of erosions becomes less critical for the diagnosis and assessment of treatment response.[24] Sonographically, erosions are defined as breaks in the bony cortex that are detected in 2 perpendicular planes (typically long and short axis).[25] Distribution and localization of erosions is the same as in radiographic findings. Marginal erosions in rheumatoid arthritis are found in proximal interphalangeal joints, metacarpophalangeal joints, wrists including distal radius and ulna, and other peripheral joints.

Table 5
Enthesitis in seronegative spondyloarthropathies

	Description	Sonographic Appearance	Rheumatic Condition
Enthesitis	Thickening and edema of tendon near insertion or origin above normal values. Hyperemia at and near interface of tendon and bone. Calcification in tendon body near attachment	Loss of densely packed hyperechoic fibrillar pattern of tendon. Hyperemia seen on Doppler ultrasonography	Seronegative spondyloarthropathies (spondyloarthritis): Psoriatic arthritis Ankylosing spondylitis Reactive arthritis Spondyloarthritis associated with inflammatory bowel disease
Enthesitis-associated bursitis		Proliferation of synovial tissue in bursae near tendon attachment. Doppler signal may be seen	Undifferentiated spondyloarthritis Juvenile enthesitis–related arthritis
Enthesitis-related bony erosion		Bony erosions at or near attachment point, outside of synovial joints	

Table 6
Detection of bony erosion by ultrasonography: break in the cortical contour of bone seen in two perpendicular planes

Rheumatic Condition	Associated Tissues	Appearance of Adjacent Bone
Rheumatoid arthritis–associated bony erosion	Associated with invading synovial pannus tissue. Therefore found within synovial joints. May occasionally be associated with tenosynovitis if pannus breaks through tendon sheath	No associated new bone formation
Osteoarthritis-associated bony erosion	No invading synovial tissue seen. Rarely synovial proliferation in adjacent capsular lumen (particularly if calcium deposits present)	Bone-spur formation is common
Gout-related bony erosion	No invading synovial tissue seen. Gouty tophi may be seen invading subchondral bone	Marginal bony overhangs are typical
Enthesitis-related erosion (see **Table 5**)	Erosions at or near enthesis, outside of synovial joint	New bone formation common

Pearls, pitfalls, and variants

Gout: double contour versus interface reflex

In gout, monosodium urate (uric acid) crystal can precipitate on hyaline cartilage over bony surfaces in joints, creating the sonographic appearance of a "double contour."[20] The hyperechoic, bright bony contour is covered by anechoic (or hypoechoic) dark hyaline cartilage. Bright, hyperechoic crystalline deposits form the second contour, which may be confounded with the bright, hyperechoic interface reflex over hyaline cartilage. This reflex is created when sound waves are reflected at the angle of perpendicular incidence off the surface of cartilage. This bright outline usually appears at the surface area of cartilage that is nearest to the transducer (if no beam steer is used). In contrast to this, the rough surface deposits of urate crystals follow the contour of the bone over a wider area. The crystal deposits create multiple small surfaces that reflect the sound waves in all directions. The reflection of the double contour sign is therefore less dependent on the angle of incidence.

Synovial hyperemia: artifact versus real signal

Ultrasonography is particularly well suited to detect and characterize inflamed tissues.[21] Power Doppler or color Doppler signals can be seen in synovial tissues of patients who would otherwise be thought to be in clinical remission based on physical examination and serology.[22] Sensitivity and specificity of Doppler signals are increased if a few simple rules are applied. Doppler signals are seen over a larger area if the overall Doppler gain is increased. With maximal gain, the entire "Doppler box" can be filled with signals. Decrease the gain until artifacts deep to the bony surface just disappear (ultrasound at frequencies used in MSK ultrasonography cannot penetrate bone; any signals that appear deep to the bony cortex are therefore artifacts by default). Keep the Doppler box small, but make sure it extends over the area of interest; this will take up less computing power and provide faster image turnover. Identify suspicious areas (eg, hypoechoic synovitis) on gray scale first. Try to match any Doppler signals with this area identified on gray scale. Making anatomic "sense" of your signals is one of the best protections against mistaking artifacts for actual blood flow. Look for Doppler signals that stay steady over the same area, and disregard signals that appear and disappear randomly. Look out for Doppler signals that are synchronous with the patient's pulse: this will be a real signal. Motion of patient or examiner will create motion artifacts; steady your hand, anchor your transducer hand at the patient or surface of desk/examination table, and use two hands to stabilize your probe, if needed. The patient's extremity should be positioned on a stable surface to help avoid Doppler motion artifacts.

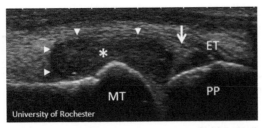

Fig. 6. Metacarpophalangeal joint 2. Radial long-axis view. Same patient as in **Fig. 7**. Power Doppler signal is seen over synovial tissue invading subchondral bone.

Invading synovial pannus tissue may be observed, and synovial hyperemia may be seen using color or power Doppler ultrasonography. In gout, "punched-out" lesions, possibly with thin marginal overhangs, can be observed radiographically and ultrasonographically. Invading tophi, but not invading synovial pannus, can be observed frequently. In erosive osteoarthritis, proximal or distal interphalangeal joints may be involved, typically with central cortical breaks.

Synovitis

Proliferative synovial tissue emanates from the synovial lining of synovial joints, lining of tendon sheath, lining of tendon body, or lining of bursae (**Fig. 8**). In joints this tissue can form an arborescent pattern, or a more plump "pannus" tissue. In inflammatory arthritis including rheumatoid arthritis and spondyloarthritis (most commonly psoriatic arthritis), this tissue can be observed invading the subchondral bone. The delicate synovial lining (1–3 cell layers strong) is not typically seen sonographically in normal controls. Proliferative synovial tissue has a hypoechoic sonographic appearance. Once detected with gray-scale ultrasonography, this tissue should be examined with

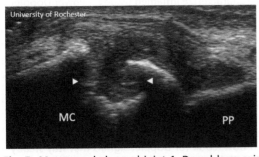

Fig. 7. Metatarsophalangeal joint 1. Dorsal long-axis view. Asterisk placed within synovial tissue. Arrow points to displaced triangular portion of joint capsule. Arrowheads denote distended joint capsule. ET, short extensor tendon inserting with joint capsule at proximal phalanx (PP); MT, metatarsal head.

color or power Doppler ultrasonography for the presence of hyperemia. Vascularization of synovial tissue detected sonographically correlates well with histologic findings after biopsy.[26] Synovial hyperemia is the strongest predictor of future joint damage in early rheumatoid arthritis.[27,28] Synovial hyperemia is also a marker of activity of arthritis that is sensitive to change. With successful treatment of inflammatory arthritis, synovial hyperemia improves first, followed by involution of synovial thickening.

Tenosynovitis

By definition, tenosynovitis can be observed only where tendons and adjacent tissue are protected from mechanical stress by sheaths. Synovial proliferation within tendon sheaths can be the earliest imaging feature of rheumatoid arthritis.[29] The fourth and sixth extensor compartments of the wrists can be used as sentinel regions for early detection of tenosynovitis in rheumatoid arthritis. Midline long-axis views over the dorsal wrists and long-axis as well as short-axis views over the extensor carpi ulnaris tendon are useful views. Look for hypoechoic, nondisplaceable tissue interposed between hyperechoic tendon sheath and hyperechoic tendon. Simple synovial fluid would be displaceable with transducer pressure. Similar to proliferation in synovial joints, tenosynovium should be examined both with gray-scale and Doppler ultrasonography. Follow-up studies can help document a treatment response.

Crystal Arthritis

Monosodium urate tophi and calcium-containing crystals can be detected sonographically. With experience, ultrasonography may replace arthrocentesis and polarizing microscopy for diagnosing gout or chondrocalcinosis in the future. Gouty tophi are strongly echogenic, often oval-shaped bodies with an anechoic rim. These tophi are commonly embedded in fibrovascular matrix tissue that may display color or power Doppler signals even in clinically asymptomatic patients. If conventional radiographs are also available, gouty tophi are seen sonographically but not radiographically. By contrast, calcium-containing crystal aggregates are typically seen both sonographically and with conventional radiography (with sonography as the slightly more sensitive imaging modality for chondrocalcinosis, in accessible joints).[30] Monosodium urate crystals may deposit on hyaline cartilage within joints. A double contour of hyperechoic bone and hyperechoic

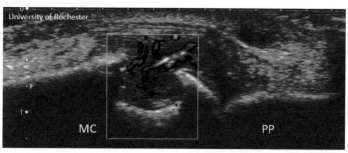

Fig. 8. Metacarpophalangeal joint 2. Radial long-axis view. Erosive arthritis. Erosion between arrowheads. MC, metacarpal head; PP, proximal phalanx.

urate deposits, separated by anechoic or hypoechoic hyaline cartilage, can be seen.

Calcium pyrophosphate is deposited in central lacunes of hyaline cartilage and fibrocartilage.[31,32] Calcium pyrophosphate deposits can therefore be distinguished from a gouty double contour by the different pattern of distribution of crystals.

Enthesitis

Enthesitis has been called a hallmark feature of seronegative spondyloarthropathies. A clinical examination can give an indication but not proof of entheseal inflammation. Both ultrasonography and contrast-enhanced MR imaging can detect enthesitis. Ultrasonography appears to be more sensitive than MR imaging.[33,34]

It may be challenging to distinguish mechanical enthesopathy from spondyloarthropathy-associated enthesitis by sonographic criteria. Enthesitis is characterized sonographically by thickening of the tendon near its proximal or distal attachment above normal values, loss of typically densely packed hyperechoic fibrillar pattern, synovial proliferation in adjacent synovial structures, hyperemia at the interface of tendon and bone, and new bone formation near the attachment point.

PRACTICAL CONSIDERATIONS

For a streamlined ultrasound examination for rheumatologic indications, it is helpful to be familiar with local regulations.

- For a screening examination of hand and wrist for rheumatoid arthritis or a similar arthropathy, will there be reimbursement for one or both extremities on the same day?
- At what intervals will follow-up examinations be reimbursed?
- Will a standardized protocol be followed?
- Will this be a comprehensive ultrasound examination of a joint area, which includes assessment of several anatomic structures, or a limited examination that focuses on a single anatomic structure?
- What are the requirements for labeling of images, report generation, transmission of report to referring provider, and storage/backup of ultrasound images?
- Are there specific requirements for the qualification of the examiner?

Helpful guidelines and protocols are provided by the European League Against Rheumatism (EULAR), the European Society of Musculoskeletal Radiology (ESSR), and the American Institute of Ultrasound in Medicine (AIUM).

For hands-on training in MSK ultrasonography in rheumatologic indications, training courses are offered by EULAR and the American College of Rheumatology (ACR). Online distance training for trainees and mentors at teaching institutions is offered through the Ultrasound School of North American Rheumatologists (www.ussonar.org).

Certification of proficiency in MSK ultrasonography for individuals can be obtained through the ACR (www.rheumatology.org). The American Registry for Diagnostic Medical Sonography also offers a certifying examination in MSK ultrasonography.

Accreditation of practices (not individual providers) can be obtained through the AIUM (www.aium.org).

SUMMARY

Ultrasonography has become an indispensable tool for the assessment of rheumatic conditions over the last 20 years. Typical erosions can be detected with greater sensitivity than with conventional radiography. Detection of synovitis, tenosynovitis, and synovial hyperemia can help with early detection of rheumatic disease and facilitate timely treatment. Serial sonography can help monitor treatment. Ineffective treatment can be modified based on ultrasonographic findings to help prevent future joint damage and potential disability. Guidance of procedures using ultrasound will lead to better accuracy, improved patient comfort, and improved clinical outcomes.

REFERENCES

1. Thiele RG. Ultrasonography applications in diagnosis and management of early rheumatoid arthritis. Rheum Dis Clin North Am 2012;38(2):259–75.
2. Scheel AK, Schmidt WA, Hermann KG, et al. Interobserver reliability of rheumatologists performing musculoskeletal ultrasonography: results from a EULAR "Train the trainers" course. Ann Rheum Dis 2005;64(7):1043–9.
3. Ohrndorf S, Naumann L, Grundey J, et al. Is musculoskeletal ultrasonography an operator-dependent method or a fast and reliably teachable diagnostic tool? Interreader agreements of three ultrasonographers with different training levels. Int J Rheumatol 2010;2010:164518.
4. Howard RNG, Pillinger MH, Gyftopoulos S, et al. Concordance between ultrasound readers determining presence of monosodium urate crystal deposition in knee and toe joints. Arthritis Rheum 2010; 62(Suppl 10):S672.
5. Ruma J, Klein KA, Chong S, et al. Cross-sectional examination interpretation discrepancies between on-call diagnostic radiology residents and subspecialty faculty radiologists: analysis by imaging modality and subspecialty. J Am Coll Radiol 2011; 8(6):409–14.
6. Mandl P, Balint PV, Brault Y, et al. Metrologic properties of ultrasound versus clinical evaluation of synovitis in rheumatoid arthritis: results of a multicenter, randomized study. Arthritis Rheum 2012;64(4): 1272–82.
7. Wakefield RJ, Gibbon WW, Conaghan PG, et al. The value of sonography in the detection of bone erosions in patients with rheumatoid arthritis: a comparison with conventional radiography. Arthritis Rheum 2000;43(12):2762–70.
8. Thiele RG. Role of ultrasound and other advanced imaging in the diagnosis and management of gout. Curr Rheumatol Rep 2011;13(2):146–53.
9. D'Agostino MA, Aegerter P, Jousse-Joulin S, et al. How to evaluate and improve the reliability of power Doppler ultrasonography for assessing enthesitis in spondylarthritis. Arthritis Rheum 2009;61(1):61–9.
10. D'Agostino MA, Said-Nahal R, Hacquard-Bouder C, et al. Assessment of peripheral enthesitis in the spondylarthropathies by ultrasonography combined with power Doppler: a cross-sectional study. Arthritis Rheum 2003;48(2):523–33.
11. Khosla S, Thiele RG, Baumhauer JF. Injection of foot and ankle joints: comparison of guidance by palpation, ultrasonography and fluoroscopy with anatomic dissection as gold standard. Arthritis Rheum 2008; 58(Suppl 9):S408.
12. Thiele RG. Musculoskeletal joint interventions. In: Dogra VS, Saad WE, editors. Ultrasound-guided procedures. New York: Thieme; 2010. p. 229–43.
13. Schmidt WA, Kraft HE, Volker L, et al. Colour Doppler sonography to diagnose temporal arteritis. Lancet 1995;345(8953):866.
14. Schmidt WA, Nerenheim A, Seipelt E, et al. Diagnosis of early Takayasu arteritis with sonography. Rheumatology (Oxford) 2002;41(5):496–502.
15. Schmidt WA, Wernicke D, Kiefer E, et al. Colour duplex sonography of finger arteries in vasculitis and in systemic sclerosis. Ann Rheum Dis 2006; 65(2):265–7.
16. Wernicke D, Hess H, Gromnica-Ihle E, et al. Ultrasonography of salivary glands—a highly specific imaging procedure for diagnosis of Sjogren's syndrome. J Rheumatol 2008;35(2):285–93.
17. McGonagle D, Benjamin M, Marzo-Ortega H, et al. Advances in the understanding of entheseal inflammation. Curr Rheumatol Rep 2002;4(6):500–6.
18. McGonagle D, Lories RJ, Tan AL, et al. The concept of a "synovio-entheseal complex" and its implications for understanding joint inflammation and damage in psoriatic arthritis and beyond. Arthritis Rheum 2007;56(8):2482–91.
19. Backhaus M, Ohrndorf S, Kellner H, et al. Evaluation of a novel 7-joint ultrasound score in daily rheumatologic practice: a pilot project. Arthritis Rheum 2009; 61(9):1194–201.
20. Thiele RG, Schlesinger N. Diagnosis of gout by ultrasound. Rheumatology (Oxford) 2007;46(7):1116–21.
21. Thiele R. Doppler ultrasonography in rheumatology: adding color to the picture. J Rheumatol 2008;35(1): 8–10.
22. Brown AK, Quinn MA, Karim Z, et al. Presence of significant synovitis in rheumatoid arthritis patients with disease-modifying antirheumatic drug-induced clinical remission: evidence from an imaging study may explain structural progression. Arthritis Rheum 2006;54(12):3761–73.
23. Thiele RG, Schlesinger N. Ultrasound detects more erosions in gout than conventional radiography. Arthritis Rheum 2010;62(Suppl 10):S368–9.

24. Schlesinger N, Thiele RG. The pathogenesis of bone erosions in gouty arthritis. Ann Rheum Dis 2010; 69(11):1907–12.

25. Wakefield RJ, Balint PV, Szkudlarek M, et al. Musculoskeletal ultrasound including definitions for ultrasonographic pathology. J Rheumatol 2005;32(12):2485–7.

26. Walther M, Harms H, Krenn V, et al. Correlation of power Doppler sonography with vascularity of the synovial tissue of the knee joint in patients with osteoarthritis and rheumatoid arthritis. Arthritis Rheum 2001;44(2):331–8.

27. Fukae J, Isobe M, Kitano A, et al. Radiographic prognosis of finger joint damage predicted by early alteration in synovial vascularity in patients with rheumatoid arthritis: potential utility of power Doppler sonography in clinical practice. Arthritis Care Res (Hoboken) 2011;63(9):1247–53.

28. Foltz V, Gandjbakhch F, Etchepare F, et al. Power Doppler ultrasound, but not low-field magnetic resonance imaging, predicts relapse and radiographic disease progression in rheumatoid arthritis patients with low levels of disease activity. Arthritis Rheum 2012;64(1):67–76.

29. Thiele RG, Tabechian D, Anandarajah AP. Ultrasonographic demonstration of tenosynovitis preceding joint involvement in early seropositive rheumatoid arthritis. Arthritis Rheum 2008;58(Suppl 9):S407.

30. Thiele RG, Schlesinger N. Ultrasound detects calcium pyrophosphate dehydrate crystal deposition in hyaline cartilage more readily than conventional radiography and MRI in pyrophosphate arthropathy. Arthritis Rheum 2007;56(Suppl 9):S1618.

31. Schumacher HR. Pathology of the synovial membrane in gout. Light and electron microscopic studies. Interpretation of crystals in electron micrographs. Arthritis Rheum 1975;18(Suppl 6):771–82.

32. Reginato AJ, Schumacher HR, Martinez VA. The articular cartilage in familial chondrocalcinosis. Light and electron microscopic study. Arthritis Rheum 1974;17(6):977–92.

33. Kamel M, Eid H, Mansour R. Ultrasound detection of heel enthesitis: a comparison with magnetic resonance imaging. J Rheumatol 2003;30(4):774–8.

34. Kamel M, Eid H, Mansour R. Ultrasound detection of knee patellar enthesitis: a comparison with magnetic resonance imaging. Ann Rheum Dis 2004;63(2):213–4.

35. Schmidt WA, Schmidt H, Schicke B, et al. Standard reference values for musculoskeletal ultrasonography. Ann Rheum Dis 2004;63(8):988–94.

Ultrasound-Guided Procedures
Soft Tissue Masses, Joints, Tendons, and Muscles

Tobias De Zordo, MD[a],*, Cesare Romagnoli, MD, FRCPC[b]

KEYWORDS

- Joints • Tendons • Muscles • Nerves • Injections • Aspiration

KEY POINTS

- US guidance of musculoskeletal interventions is easy to perform, relatively inexpensive, widely available, and minimally invasive.
- Basic knowledge of anatomy is fundamental for accurate US guidance to avoid neurovascular structures.
- High-resolution US equipment should be used for exact needle placement in all musculoskeletal interventions.
- All procedures require proper training under supervision at the beginning, but fast learning curves are reported.

 Videos of ultrasound application to cyst injection; fragmentation and aspiration of calcific tendinosis; aspiration of masses; and foreign body removal accompany this article.

INTRODUCTION

Ultrasound (US) guidance for musculoskeletal interventions has become more and more popular over recent decades. US is the first-line imaging tool for musculoskeletal disorders providing excellent image quality of muscles, tendons, and joints. High-resolution US equipment with frequencies of up to 20 MHz can be used allowing for best resolution in superficially located structures, such as the musculoskeletal system. For musculoskeletal interventions high-resolution US is mostly superior to computed tomography (CT) or magnetic resonance imaging (MRI). Its ready availability has led to widespread use of US guidance in musculoskeletal interventions. US is radiation free, less expensive, and faster than CT or MRI, and more accurate than clinical guidance alone. US guidance allows accurate placement of the needle with real-time visualization of the procedure. Correct needle placement is crucial in musculoskeletal disorders to allow for aspiration or for successful injections. In comparison with blind procedures, US guidance has been shown to significantly improve the accuracy of joint aspiration and injection.[1] In blind interventions correct needle placement fails in up to 75% and is most difficult in small joints and tendons.[2]

Common indications for US guidance in musculoskeletal disorders include aspiration of fluids in joints or tendons; injection of corticosteroids in joints, bursae, or tendon sheaths; and soft tissue biopsies. Other therapeutic interventions are perforation and lavage of tendon calcifications; removal of foreign bodies; hyaluronic acid injections in joints; dry needling or autologous blood injections in tendinopathy; or prolotheraphy, which is a hyperosmolar dextrose injection into a tendon sheath. US

[a] Department of Radiology, Medical University Innsbruck, Anichstr. 35, 6020 Innsbruck, Tyrol, Austria;
[b] Department of Medical Imaging, Robarts Research Institute, University of Western Ontario, 100 Perth Dr, London, ON, N6A 5K8, Canada
* Corresponding author.
E-mail address: Tobias@De-Zordo.net

Ultrasound Clin 7 (2012) 537–550
http://dx.doi.org/10.1016/j.cult.2012.08.007
1556-858X/12/$ – see front matter © 2012 Elsevier Inc. All rights reserved.

guidance can also be routinely used for injection of contrast agents in CT or MR arthrography.

This article discusses technical and pharmacologic aspects, describes different musculoskeletal interventions, and delineates the different approaches according to anatomic structures.

TECHNICAL CONSIDERATIONS
US Hardware and Settings

The main advantage of US-guided interventions lies in the fact that the needle position can be visualized in real-time and therefore direct visualization of the procedure is possible when high-end US systems are used. High-resolution US equipment is crucial when performing US-guided musculoskeletal interventions. US frequencies of 5 MHz or higher should be used depending on the anatomic location: in spine, hip, or obese patients, less than 7 MHz; in shoulder, elbow, knee, and ankle joints, 7 to 18 MHz; in finger and toe joints, hockey stick probes are available with frequencies up to 18 MHz; and in muscles and tendons located superficially the highest possible frequencies should be applied.

Before performing an intervention detailed assessment of the pathology has to be performed and images should be recorded. For best image quality individual optimization of US frequency, depth, focus, and gain is fundamental and should be performed before the intervention. Documentation of the intervention can be performed by saving video clips or at least by showing correct needle placement on a single image.

Instrumentation

For all musculoskeletal interventions strict sterile handling is necessary. The area of interest should be disinfected and the surrounding region draped. The US transducer should be disinfected with alcohol 70% or a chlorhexidine solution and covered with a sterile sheath. Sterile US gel or proviodine can be used to guarantee skin-probe contact, and sterile gloves should be worn.

Next, the pathology should be visualized and a viable needle path should be identified. The entrance point at the skin can be marked with a sterile marker. Needle size is chosen according to the procedure. For injections of anesthetics or corticosteroids smaller-size needles ($\geq$21 gauge) are mostly sufficient, whereas in interventions where fluid aspiration or destruction of calcifications is performed larger-bore needles are used (16–21 gauge). For biopsy, the needle size is 20 to 14 gauge.

For all musculoskeletal procedures we prefer a free-hand needle technique to allow for flexible positioning of the needle during the intervention.

When the transducer is oriented longitudinally along the same plane as the needle track axis, the needle appears as a bright echogenic linear structure, often showing a posterior ring down artifact. Alternatively, positioning the transducer transverse to the needle depicts the needle as a bright echogenic dot. Gently wobbling the needle or injecting a small amount of anesthetic or saline and observing the moving echoes may assist in identifying the needle position.[3]

For all interventions an assistant is needed to allow for sterile handling.

Pharmacologic Aspects

Local anesthesia is only necessary when large-bore needles are used and when painful procedures, such as needling, are performed. We use lidocaine 1% for local anesthesia, which can also be used for diagnostic injections of joints without significant adverse effects.[4] Most of the time the patient experiences a mild or moderate burning sensation. Bicarbonate (1 mL) might be added before loading the lidocaine into the syringe, which helps to prevent the burning sensation.

For US-guided injections of MR contrast agents a mixture of 1:200 (gadolinium/saline) is generally used. Depending on the joint a volume from 2 mL (wrist) to 15 mL (shoulder) might be injected.

When performing therapeutic injections with corticosteroids we always use soluble corticosteroid for tendons, whereas for joint injections soluble or crystalline suspension of corticosteroids can be used. Crystalline suspensions (eg, dexamethasone) have the advantage that their effects last longer (up to 3 months), which is especially useful in patients with rheumatoid disorders. In patients with traumatic disorders we prefer a shorter lasting (weeks) soluble corticosteroid (eg, betamethasone). Indications for corticosteroid injections have to be checked carefully because a chondrotoxic effect of such treatment was described.[5]

The injected volume is normally between 1 mL for small joints and 10 mL for larger joints, such as the knee. It should always be based on the patient's sensation; when patients describe pain after injection maximal tension of the joint capsule might be present and injection should be interrupted.

Adverse Reactions and Complications

Although complications are uncommon, possible adverse affects of musculoskeletal interventions include the following:

- Local bruising
- Minor bleeding

- Seldom loss of pigment in the skin that was entered by the needle
- Aspiration or injections of anesthetics into the musculoskeletal system does not do any harm by itself, but may cause the most serious complication, which is infection especially of joints; therefore, aseptic conditions are absolutely indispensable[6]

When injecting corticosteroids adverse effects include:

- Erythemal responses
- Swelling at the injection site
- Inflammation of a joint caused by the crystalline substance
- Atrophy of the subcutaneous fat tissue
- Loss of skin pigmentation
- Systemic complications are rarely encountered and include aggravation of diabetes mellitus by increase in blood sugar, and exacerbation of preexisting infections in other organs
- Multiple injections of corticosteroids may lead to systemic side effects, such as weight gain, puffy face and trunk, and easy bruising. Therefore, we recommend injecting corticosteroids not more than four to six times a year.[6]

INTERVENTIONS
Aspiration

Fluid aspiration from joints is performed for diagnostic and therapeutic causes. Analysis of joint fluid can help to diagnose causes of joint swelling or arthritis, such as infection, gout, pseudogout, or rheumatic disease. Joint fluid can be tested for white cell count, crystals, protein, and glucose, and cultured to detect bacterial infection and in rare cases to detect malignancy.

All fluid aspirations are also therapeutic; swelling of joints, bursae (**Fig. 1**), or tendon sheaths because of fluid causes pain. Therefore, especially aspirations of large fluid collections give the patient relief. However, it has to be taken into account that aspiration of fluid is only a symptomatic treatment and the cause of the disease is not treated (**Fig. 2**).[6]

Fluid collections may occur in muscles, representing in most cases hematomas. Acute hematomas are easily detectable by US and can be aspirated under US guidance when necessary. However, aspiration should not be performed in an acute setting to avoid rebleeding, and in most cases hematomas are reabsorbed after a few days to weeks. We perform aspiration of hematomas only in chronic cases to assist the healing process. Sometimes, when the hematoma becomes chronic, it can mimic a semisolid mass with septa and hyperemic structures. In such cases biopsy of the solid-appearing structures can be performed to rule out malignancy.[6]

Arthrography

MR and CT arthrography are well-proved and useful techniques for the diagnosis of intra-articular lesions. At the shoulder, glenoid labrum, glenohumeral ligaments, and the intra-articular portion of the rotator cuff tendons can be accurately assessed.[7] At the hip, CT and MR arthrography allow the precise diagnosis of labral tears; loose bodies; and intra-articular ligaments (capsular and ligamentum teres).[8] Less commonly arthrography is used for assessing the wrist, elbow, knee, or ankle.

MR and CT arthrography require previous injection of contrast agents into the joints. Although it is commonly reported to be performed under fluoroscopic guidance, US guidance is becoming more

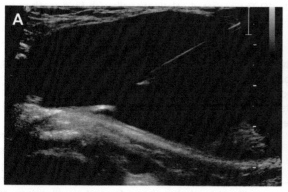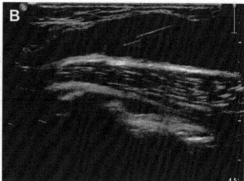

Fig. 1. (*A*) Large Baker cyst. US-guided introduction of an 18-G spinal needle for aspiration. (*B*) Same patient after aspiration of about 20 mL of clear, yellowish fluid under direct control of ultrasound. Aspiration was followed by injection of steroid and ropivicaine.

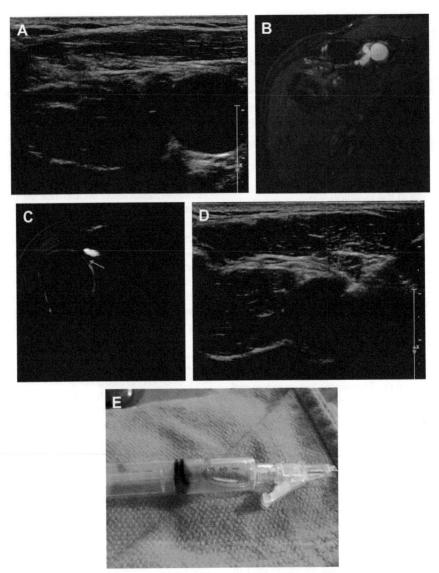

Fig. 2. (*A*) B-mode US before intervention: ganglion cyst in the supraspinatus fossa of the right shoulder. (*B*) Corresponding MRI image of the same patient showing a ganglion cyst at the right shoulder. (*C*) MRI of the same patient reveals a ganglion cyst caused by a tear of the superior labrum (*arrow*). (*D*) Aspiration of the paralabral ganglion cyst under US guidance using a 16-G needle. (*E*) The aspirated gelatinous yellowish fluid confirms the diagnosis of a ganglion cyst.

and more popular because of its wide availability and lack of radiation.[7,9] US-guided injection for MR arthrography represents a simple, safe, and effective technique that yields comparable results to those of injection under fluoroscopic guidance, but is slightly more time-consuming.[9]

Therapeutic Injection

US-guided injection of corticosteroids into joints, tendons, or bursae (**Fig. 3**) (video 1) is one of the most common indications in musculoskeletal interventions. Overuse of joints, tendons, or bursae, degenerative disease, or rheumatoid disorders cause fluid accumulation, hypervascularization, and synovial proliferation (**Fig. 4**), which can be easily treated with local injections.

The mechanism of corticosteroid action includes a reduction of the inflammatory reaction by limiting the capillary dilatation and permeability of the vascular structures.[10] When injection without aspiration is performed needle sizes of up to 26 gauge only can be used. Smaller-sized needles are better tolerated by patients and cause

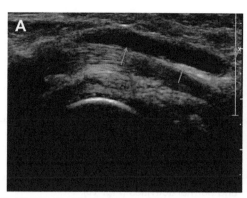
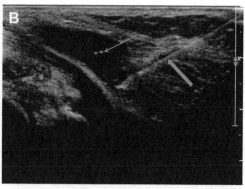

Fig. 3. (*A*) B-mode US shows a small Baker cyst in the popliteal fossa of the right knee (*arrows*). (*B*) Injection of steroid and ropivicaine using a 25-G needle (*thick arrow*) was performed under US guidance. The presence of tiny gas bubbles (*thin arrow*) spreading inside the cyst confirms that the injection is successful.

less damage to the surrounding soft tissue. Care has to be taken to avoid injection of corticosteroids in previously inflamed areas, which may result in acute exacerbation of the inflammation causing sepsis and perhaps death.

Of special concern are injections of corticosteroids in tendons: US guidance is crucial in such cases to avoid intratendinous injections (**Fig. 5**). The tip of the needle has to be clearly identified in the tendon sheath and only then should injection of fluid corticosteroids be performed (**Fig. 6**). Crystalline corticosteroids should be omitted when treating tendons to avoid abrading the tendon, possibly resulting in partial or complete tear of the already damaged tendon.[11]

Newer research is focusing on injections of hyaluronic acids into arthritic joints (**Fig. 7**). Although initial results have shown good results for large joints, such as the knee and hip, only a few studies are available and further research has to be performed.[12] Another interesting field of research

is so-called "prolotherapy," where dextrose injection into tendons is supposed to cause faster healing.[13] However, even for this technique further studies have to clarify the therapeutic effect and long-term studies are in demand.

Another recently developed therapeutic option is autologous blood injection into tendinopatic alterations, with very good results.[14] Although cultivation of blood cells is time consuming and cost expensive, preliminary results show good success rates. A less complicated but similar technique is called "needling." Under US guidance repeated puncturing of a tendon insertion or origin causes aseptic inflammation resulting in a faster healing response.[15]

Foreign Body Extraction

US is able to detect foreign bodies and can be used to guide foreign body extraction (video 2). US-guided removal of superficial foreign bodies

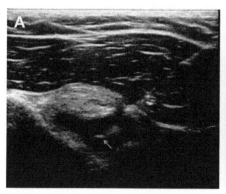
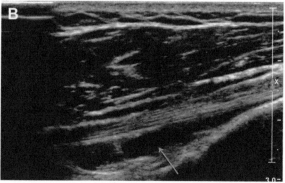

Fig. 4. (*A*) Axial view of the long head of the biceps tendon (*star*) during US-guided tendon sheath injection. The tip of the needle (*arrow*) should be positioned in between the tendon and the bony surface. (*B*) Longitudinal view of the long head of the biceps tendon after injection. The increased amount of fluid within the tendon sheath confirms the injection was placed correctly in the tendon sheath (*arrow*).

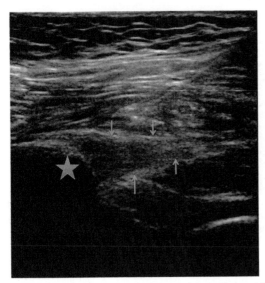

Fig. 5. Longitudinal view during injection of steroid and marcaine 0.5% at the anteroinferior iliac spine (*star*) along the rectus femoris tendon (*arrows*).

can be performed more easily when the composition of the fragment is metallic or gravel. Removal of glass or wooden splinters requires more patience and meticulous technique. Besides adequate local anesthesia, a set of sterilized surgical instruments, including Mosquito, Kelly, Kocher, and Splinter forceps, is needed. After marking the position of the best extractable side, a skin incision is necessary to allow for instrumentation. Real-time US guidance visualizes the entire procedure, resulting in an accurate, simpler, and less invasive removal of a splinter compared with open surgery (**Fig. 8**).[6]

Treatment of Calcific Tendinitis

Calcific tendinitis is caused by calcium hydroxyapatite deposition in tendons. Predominately the rotator cuff tendons are involved with a higher incidence in women. Although calcific tendinitis is a self-limiting process, in about 50% patients become symptomatic. The clinical history of calcific tendinosis includes two phases: the formative phase can last years and involves progressive accumulation of "solid" calcium within the tendon, causing a small or moderate amount of pain, with some degree of decreased range of motion (**Fig. 9**). The resorptive phase usually lasts weeks or months. The calcium becomes "soft" or like "toothpaste." The patient usually experiences excruciating pain, with severe limitation of motion and normal activities (**Fig. 10**).

US-guided puncture and lavage is one of the most promising treatment options when patients complain of acute or chronic pain. After local anesthesia, the calcification is punctured with a 16-gauge needle under US guidance to fragment the calcific deposits (video 3). In the next step we insert a second needle and, while saline is injected through the first needle, aspiration of the cloudy, milky, or solid gritty substance is performed through the second needle (**Fig. 11**, video 4).[16] Other authors describe a single needle procedure, where they inject and aspirate through the same needle. During aspiration different results can be achieved: (1) toothpaste material when the calcium is in the resorptive phase (**Fig. 12**), (2) tiny calcific fragments in the formative phase, (3) milk of calcium fluid, and (4) in a not insignificant number of cases nothing is aspirated. This is not a sign of failure of the procedure, because the fragmentation and the saline injection cause the mobilization of the calcium into the subdeltoid bursa, followed by absorption, virtually in every case.[17]

In most cases only a part of the calcification can be aspirated, but the residual calcification tends to undergo spontaneous mobilization into the subdeltoid bursa and then resorption. The presence of calcium in the subdeltoid bursa irritates the synovial lining and could cause significant pain. Before extraction of the needle, intrabursal

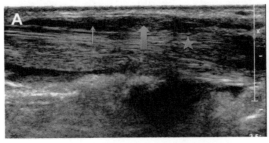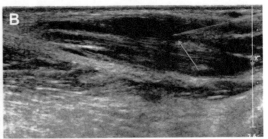

Fig. 6. (*A*) Longitudinal B-mode US view of the peroneal tendons (*star*) with fluid (*thin arrow*) and a synovial nodule (*thick arrow*) in the tendon sheath before intervention. (*B*) US-guided injection of corticosteroid and marcaine 0.5% around the peroneal tendons. Direct visualization of the needle's tip (*arrow*) is crucial to avoid intratendinous placement of corticosteroids possibly causing tendon rupture.

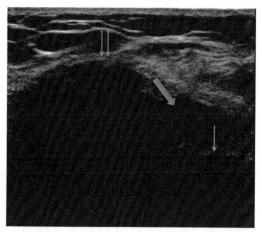

Fig. 7. Hyaluronic acid (Neovisc) injection of knee. US guidance is helpful in overweight or obese patients. The needle (*thick arrow*) is carefully inserted between the patella (*double arrow*) and the femoral condyle (*single arrow*).

injection of corticosteroids and long-acting anesthetics is suggested to decrease crystal-induced inflammation. In most cases this is good enough to protect the patient. In a significant minority of cases the protection fades before the absorption of calcium is completed. This happens more likely when a large amount of calcium is present. We always warn the patient that if they have significant recurrent pain after 10 to 15 days they should call to schedule a second bursal injection. A second or, rarely, a third procedure might be required when the calcific deposit is quite large.

Conventional radiographs are more reliable than US for treatment follow-up, because US cannot easily distinguish scarring from residual calcium deposit (**Fig. 13**).

Biopsy of Soft Tissue Masses

For biopsies of masses located in muscles, subcutaneous tissue, skin, joint, and tendon sheaths (**Fig. 14**) two possible approaches can be used. In aspiration for cytology, a spinal needle (22–26 G) is introduced into the mass, and fragmentation of tissue with limited bleeding is obtained with back and forth movement of the needle inside the mass (video 5). It is important to limit the bleeding, because an excessive presence of blood in the specimen can significantly impair the interpretation. It is less traumatic than a core biopsy, but

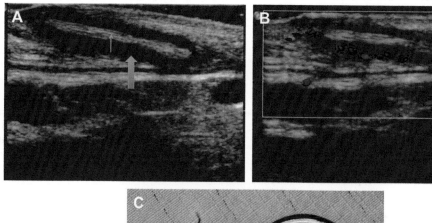

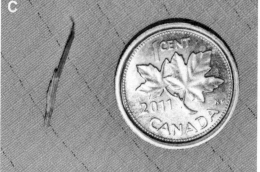

Fig. 8. (*A*) Submandibular subcutaneous foreign body (*thin arrow*) surrounded by fluid and inflammatory reaction (*thick arrow*). (*B*) Submandibular subcutaneous foreign body. Doppler US showing increased vascular flow surrounding the foreign body as sign of inflammatory reaction. (*C*) US-guided foreign body extraction was performed revealing a small splinter after removal.

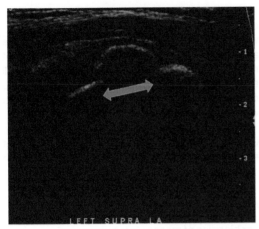

Fig. 9. "Hard" calcification of supraspinatus tendon with posterior shadowing on US (*left-right arrow*).

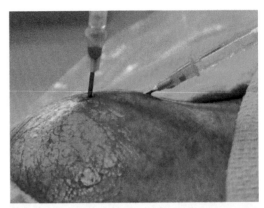

Fig. 11. Two-needle technique for lavage of calcific tendinosis. One needle is used to inject saline and the second needle to aspirate the saline solution along with calcium.

usually the characterization is limited to the dichotomy benign or malignant.

The other approach is core biopsies using biopsy guns (that sometime are disposable) with a larger diameter (gauge 16–20) (**Fig. 15**). When the mass is mobile it is important to "hook" the mass before the shooting to avoid forward displacement of the mass. It is a more aggressive procedure, but most of the time allows a more specific diagnosis.

Every time we deal with possible malignancy, seeding along the needle path is of concern. Care should be taken to avoid trespassing different compartments or, if it is not possible to discuss the biopsy strategy with the surgeon, not to jeopardize limb salvage.

APPROACHES FOR US-GUIDED INTERVENTIONS

The general technique for US-guided interventions is similar for muscles, tendons, joints, and nerves.

Patient positioning should accommodate the patient's and the physician's comfort, thus optimizing the outcome of the procedure.[3] Careful selection of the injection side is of importance because knowledge of the surrounding anatomic structures is indispensable. The needle path has to be chosen to avoid nerves and vessels and continuous visualization of the needle's tip if recommended. Injections in the vicinity of arteries should be avoided.

Shoulder

For MR arthrography patients are placed in the supine position, with external rotation of the arm. Guided by US the needle is introduced through the rotator interval space, using the humeral head and coracoid process as anatomic landmarks, immediately above the subscapularis tendon. The cortex of the humeral head is identified as a circular line in a lateral position and the

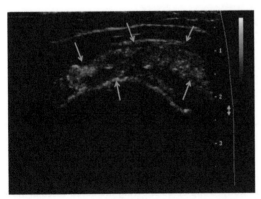

Fig. 10. Large, soft, "toothpaste" calcification (*arrows*) in the supraspinatus tendon.

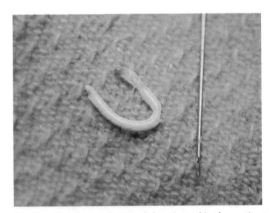

Fig. 12. "Toothpaste" material aspirated in the patient showing a "soft" calcification (see **Fig. 10**).

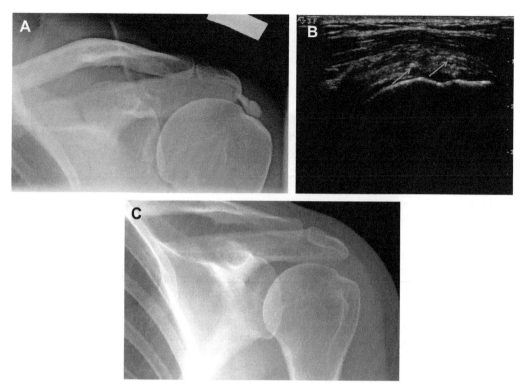

Fig. 13. (A) Radiograph showing a "solid" calcification of the supraspinatus tendon before intervention. (B) After US-guided needling and lavage scattered hyperechoic foci were present (*arrows*). US is not able to differentiate between residual calcifications and scarring. (C) Radiograph shows complete resolution of the calcific deposit. Plain films help to distinguish residual disease from scarring.

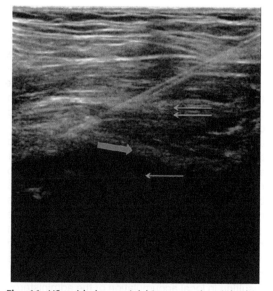

Fig. 14. US-guided synovial biopsy at the right hip. Synovial thickening (*thick arrow*) is seen between the muscle belly (*double arrow*) and the joint fluid (*single arrow*).

coracoid process as a small inverted U-shape structure medially, both echogenic and with strong posterior acoustic shadowing.[7]

For therapeutic injections the same approach can be used, but because fluid tends to accumulate first in the posterior aspect of the glenohumeral joint, a posterior approach through the infraspinatus muscle with the patient sitting or in a semiprone position should be used.[18] The needle passes into the joint space immediately deep to the free margin of the glenoid labrum and tangential to the curvature of the humeral head.[19] Glenohumeral joint injection is mainly performed in osteoarthritis; adhesive capsulitis ("frozen shoulder"); and rheumatoid arthritis.[20] Relative contraindications of glenohumeral joint injections are avascular necrosis of the humeral head and recent rotator cuff tendon rupture.[19]

Injection of corticosteroids into the subacromial-subdeltoid bursa for the treatment of bursitis, rotator cuff tendinitis, and impingement syndrome is another common and useful procedure equivalent to systemic steroid injections.[21] An anterior or lateral approach with the patient sitting or supine is recommended, with real-time visualization of the needle in a parallel position.[22] Blind

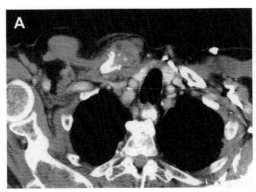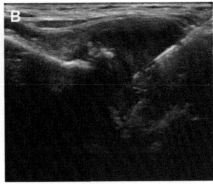

Fig. 15. (*A*) Contrast-enhanced chest CT showing a bone metastasis from adenocarcinoma at the medial aspect of the right clavicle. (*B*) US-guided core biopsy of the bone metastasis was performed.

injection is reported to fail in up to 71%.[23] Therefore, US guidance is crucial for correct placement to improve therapeutic effectiveness.[24] This procedure can also be used diagnostically to differentiate between local and referred pain.

US-guided injection is further used for treatment of inflammation of the long head of the biceps tendon[25] (see **Fig. 6**). Care has to be taken to place the tip of the needle inside the tendon sheath but not in the tendon itself.

The second shoulder joint, the acromioclavicular joint, is frequently injected in osteoarthritis. A superior approach with the patient supine or sitting is most feasible and visualization of the needle is possible by an axial view.[22]

Elbow

US-guided interventions of the elbow are required in osteoarthritis or rheumatologic diseases. The cubital joint may be punctured from a posterior approach allowing access to the olecranon recess when a large amount of fluid is present or anterolaterally through the radiocapitellar joint.[26,27] With the elbow flexed at 90 degrees the olecranon recess can be easily accessed laterally or medially from the triceps tendon or direct injection of the joint can be performed through the extensor tendons and the radiocapitellar joint.[22]

Inflammatory changes of the common extensor tendons at the lateral epicondyle ("tennis elbow") or common flexor tendons at the medial epicondyle ("golfer's elbow") are common indications for US-guided therapy. Although superficially located, US guidance can be used for peritendinous injection to avoid intratendinous placement of corticosteroids. Alternative to corticosteroids-steroids, "dry needling" (needle tenotomy) or intratendinous autologous blood injections or platelete rich plasma injections are described in the literature.[14,15,28,29]

Hand and Wrist

Osteoarthritis and rheumatoid arthritis are the most common causes of joint inflammation at the hand and wrist. The radiocarpal joint is injected through a dorsal approach about 1 to 2 cm distal to the Lister tubercle, between the second-third or third-fourth extensor tendon compartment so that needle placement through tendon sheaths and small vessels can be avoided.[30] Additional distal radioulnar joint injections should be performed when fluid or synovial proliferation is present.[22]

Intercarpal, metacarpophalangeal, proximal, and distal interphanlangeal joints are typically affected by rheumatoid arthritis, osteoarthritis, and psoriatic arthritis.[31,32] A dorsal oblique approach, laterally or medially of the extensor tendon, using a hockey stick probe allows for an easy and safe pathway with correct needle placement. Fluid accumulations are normally very small in these joints and therefore injection by real-time US guidance is recommended.[22]

Tenovaginitis of extensor or flexor tendons at the hand and wrist are often associated with overuse syndromes, but also with rheumatologic disorders, such as rheumatoid arthritis and psoriatic arthritis. US-guided fluid aspirations and therapeutic injections should be performed after accurate inspection of the tendon structure to rule out tendon rupture. The affected tendon is best approached first longitudinally and when the needle tip is placed into the tendon sheath the axial plane verifies correct needle placement. If needle placement is correct, the injection should result in distension of the sheath; however, this can be compromised by tendon sheath adhesions, resulting in local accumulation of the administered drug.[22]

Perineural injections are often performed in compression neuropathy, such as carpal tunnel syndrome. Similar to tendon procedures, longitudinal parallel scans of the needle path are performed and axial views to ascertain correct needle location have to be performed. A 27-gauge needle is placed parallel to the probe and the carpal tunnel entered, whereas the optimal entrance point is located between the medial nerve and the flexor carpi radialis tendon.[33] Care should be taken not to inject the nerve itself because this may lead to dysesthesia and nerve damage.[22]

Hip

Fluid accumulations caused by inflammatory arthritis, osteoarthritis, or after hip prosthesis are common indications for US-guided interventions at the hip.[26] With the patient in supine position an anterolateral access under the inguinal ligament toward the anterior synovial recess at the junction of the femoral head and neck should be chosen.[34] A slight increase in resistance is appreciated as the needle passes the iliofemoral ligament, but direct injection in the ligament should be avoided. With further advance, the needle can be felt to pop through the ligament and enter the hip joint.[22] Avoiding large vessels and nerves is of major importance at this localization. For MR arthography, basically the same approach can be chosen, but it might be more challenging because fluid collections are not always present.

US-guided injection of the greater trochanteric bursa or the iliopsoas tendon bursa is recommended especially in overuse syndromes. The trochanteric bursae are best approached with the patient lying on the side in the lateral decubitus position with the symptomatic side uppermost.[35] In pathologic conditions fluid accumulates inside the bursa and US guidance allows easy access to the enlarged bursa. In chronic overuse snapping of the iliopsoas tendon over the iliopectineal eminence may result in bursitis. With the probe oriented along the femoral neck, the iliopsoas tendon can be seen

lateral to the neurovascular bundle.[35] With the patient in supine position a lateral access to avoid neurovascular structures is preferred.[36]

Knee

US-guided interventions of the knee are mostly requested in patients with synovitis or fluid accumulation caused by osteoarthritis or rheumatologic disorders. Occasionally, there is periarticular ganglion cysts or pathology of the Hoffa pad (**Fig. 16**). Curtiss and colleagues[13] determined that US-guided knee injections using a superolateral approach were 100% accurate, whereas the accuracy of blind knee injections varied considerably depending on the clinician's experience. Knee-joint inflammation usually leads to fluid collection in the suprapatellar recess.

The patient is positioned supine and with the knee angulated 20 to 30 degrees, the needle is inserted from the lateral aspect of the quadriceps tendon, at the patellar insertion, directly into the fluid collection (**Fig. 17**). If the recess is not discernible on US the needle can be placed in the joint cavity, but with this traditional approach the needle is covered by bone (see **Fig. 7**) and intra-articular placement can only be detected by injecting air inside the joint cavity, which moves to the suprapatellar recess, thus making it visible.[22,34]

When a symptomatic Baker cyst with functional limitation of the knee, inflammation, rupture of the cyst, or compression of the surrounding structures is present, a dorsal approach is required.[22] US guidance is of special interest when a septated, multilobulated Baker cyst is present.[6]

Patella and popliteal tendons are often involved in overuse or traumatic injuries of the knee. Besides peritendinous corticosteroid injections newer treatment options include dry needling; autologous blood injection[14]; and hyperosmolar dextrose injections (prolotherapy).[37] US-guided

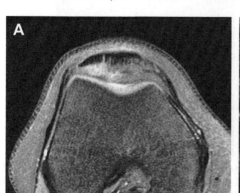
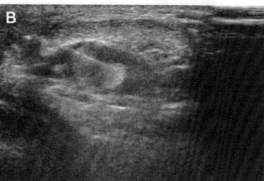

Fig. 16. (*A*) Axial MRI of the knee showing soft tissue edema in the Hoffa space, consistent with infrapatellar fat pad impingement. (*B*) US-guided injection of Hoffa fat pad using a 25-G needle.

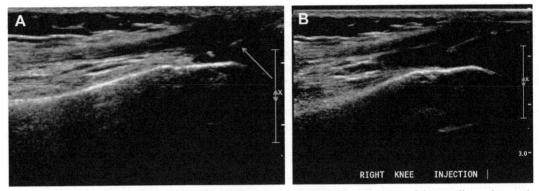

Fig. 17. (*A*) Knee injection. The presence of a small joint effusion at the lateral aspect of the patella, and posterior to the lateral retinaculum, allows a safe introduction of the needle (*arrow*) into the joint space. (*B*) The progression of the injection can be easily followed in real-time under US.

injection of the superficial patellar tendon is easy to perform by longitudinal and axial views. For the more complex injection of the popliteal tendon the patient is positioned in a lateral decubitus position with the limb flexed to 20 to 30 degrees and the leg slightly internally rotated. The popliteus tendon appears within the popliteus sulcus of the lateral femoral condyle on axial views and

by rotating the transducer a longitudinal view of the proximal tendon around the posterior aspect of the lateral femoral condyle can be obtained.[38]

Ankle and Feet

Osteoarthritis and rheumatoid disease are the most relevant indications for joint injections at

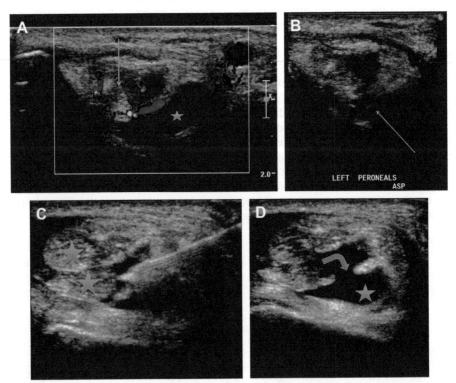

Fig. 18. (*A*) Doppler US. Synovial cyst (*star*) abutting the tendon sheath of the peroneal tendons (*arrow*), which show inflammatory reaction. (*B*) Aspiration under US guidance of the synovial cyst. Two milliliters of yellow, thickened fluid were aspirated until complete resolution. *Arrow* shows the tip of the needle. (*C*) Consequently, US-guided injection of fluid corticosteroids into the peroneal tendon (*stars*) sheath was performed. (*D*) Postinjection refilling of the synovial cyst (*star*) through a discontinuity of the tendon sheath (*curved arrow*) was observed.

the ankle or foot. At the ankle the tibiotalar, subtalar, or talonavicular joint space can be best visualized by an anterior approach after visualizing the anterior tibial artery.[39] Effusions of the ankle joint are sometimes localized exclusively in the dorsal region of the ankle joint.[40] In the latter case, the needle can be introduced from the lateral or medial side anterior to the Achilles tendon while the patient is in the prone position and the probe held in a short axis to the Achilles tendon.[40]

The intertarsal, talometatarsal, metatarsophalangeal, and interphalangeal joints are easily approached by a dorsal access. US allows one to identify the pathologic condition and the best needle pathway by avoiding tendons, nerves, and vessels.[39]

Tendons, such as Achilles, plantar fascia, flexor hallucis longus, peroneus, and tibialis, are commonly involved in overuse or traumatic or systemic diseases and injections should be performed as described for other tendons with visualization of the needle's tip in two planes to avoid intratendinous injection (**Fig. 18**).

SUMMARY

A wide variability of US-guided procedures are available and allow minimal invasive treatment of musculoskeletal disorders. Besides the conventional fluid aspiration and injection techniques, recently new therapeutic options, such as puncture and lavage of clacific tendinitis, needeling of tendons, autologous blood injections in tendons, and hyaluronic acid injection in osteoarthritis, are becoming more popular. Although long-term studies are still in demand for some of these new procedures, US guidance is crucial to allow for accurate needle placement and consequently best outcome.

SUPPLEMENTARY DATA

Videos related to this article can be found online at http://dx.doi.org/10.1016/j.cult.2012.08.007.

What the referring physician needs to know

- Collaboration with the referring physician is crucial for all musculoskeletal interventions.

- The referring physician should be aware of all possible advantages, but also of the limitation of US-guided procedures. Especially, worst case scenarios with bacterial joint inflammation or tendon rupture after injections have to be extensively discussed with the patient.

- A close collaboration is of special concern in soft tissue masses to discuss the needle pathway in case of possible seeding.

REFERENCES

1. Sibbitt WL Jr, Peisajovich A, Michael AA, et al. Does sonographic needle guidance affect the clinical outcome of intraarticular injections? J Rheumatol 2009;36:1892–902.
2. Cunnington J, Marshall N, Hide G, et al. A randomized, double-blind, controlled study of ultrasound-guided corticosteroid injection into the joint of patients with inflammatory arthritis. Arthritis Rheum 2010;62:1862–9.
3. Joines MM, Motamedi K, Seeger LL, et al. Musculoskeletal interventional ultrasound. Semin Musculoskelet Radiol 2007;11:192–8.
4. Erden IA, Altinel S, Saricaoglu F, et al. Effect of intraarticular injection of levobupivacaine on articular cartilage and synovium in rats. Anaesthesist 2012; 61:420–3.
5. Braun HJ, Wilcox-Fogel N, Kim HJ, et al. The effect of local anesthetic and corticosteroid combinations on chondrocyte viability. Knee Surg Sports Traumatol Arthrosc 2011. http://dx.doi.org/10.1007/s00167-011-1728-1.
6. Romagnoli C, De Zordo T, Klauser AS, et al. Ultrasound guided procedures. In: Dogra V, Gaitini D, editors. Musculoskeletal ultrasound with MRI and CT correlation. New York: Thieme; 2010. p. 220–43.
7. Souza PM, Aguiar RO, Marchiori E, et al. Arthrography of the shoulder: a modified ultrasound guided technique of joint injection at the rotator interval. Eur J Radiol 2010;74:e29–32.
8. Llopis E, Fernandez E, Cerezal L. MR and CT arthrography of the hip. Semin Musculoskelet Radiol 2012;16:42–56.
9. Schaeffeler C, Brügel M, Waldt S, et al. Ultrasound-guided intraarticular injection for MR arthrography of the shoulder. Rofo 2010;182:267–73.
10. Salinas JD Jr. Corticosteroid injections of joints and soft tissues. 2011. Available at: http://emedicine.medscape.com/article/325370-overview#aw2aab6b4. Accessed June 20, 2012.
11. Tempfer H, Gehwolf R, Lehner C, et al. Effects of crystalline glucocorticoid triamcinolone acetonide on cultured human supraspinatus tendon cells. Acta Orthop 2009;80:357–62.
12. Colen S, Haverkamp D, Mulier M, et al. Hyaluronic acid for the treatment of osteoarthritis in all joints except the knee: what is the current evidence? BioDrugs 2012;26:101–12.
13. Curtiss HM, Finnoff JT, Peck E, et al. Accuracy of ultrasound-guided and palpation-guided knee injections by an experienced and less-experienced injector using a superolateral approach: a cadaveric study. PM R 2011;3:507–15.
14. James SL, Ali K, Pocock C, et al. Ultrasound guided dry needling and autologous blood injection for patellar tendinosis. Br J Sports Med 2007;41:518–21.

15. Housner JA, Jacobson JA, Misko R. Sonographically guided percutaneous needle tenotomy for the treatment of chronic tendinosis. J Ultrasound Med 2009; 28:1187–92.

16. De Zordo T, Ahmad N, Ødegaard F, et al. US-guided therapy of calcific tendinopathy: clinical and radiological outcome assessment in shoulder and non-shoulder tendons. Ultraschall Med 2011;32:S117–23.

17. Sconfienza LM, Bandirali M, Serafini G, et al. Rotator cuff calcific tendinitis: does warm saline solution improve the short-term outcome of double-needle US-guided treatment? Radiology 2012;262:560–6.

18. Schmidt WA, Schicke B, Krause A. Which ultrasound scan is the best to detect glenohumeral joint effusions? Ultraschall Med 2008;29:250–5.

19. Zwar RB, Read JW, Noakes JB. Sonographically guided glenohumeral joint injection. AJR Am J Roentgenol 2004;183:48–50.

20. Tallia AF, Cardone DA. Diagnostic and therapeutic injection of the shoulder region. Am Fam Physician 2003;67:1271–8.

21. Ekeberg OM, Bautz-Holter E, Tveitå EK, et al. Subacromial ultrasound guided or systemic steroid injection for rotator cuff disease: randomised double blind study. BMJ 2009;23(338):3112.

22. De Zordo T, Mur E, Bellmann-Weiler R, et al. US guided injections in arthritis. Eur J Radiol 2009;71: 197–203.

23. Esenyel CZ, Esenyel M, Yeşiltepe R, et al. The correlation between the accuracy of steroid injections and subsequent shoulder pain and function in subacromial impingement syndrome. Acta Orthop Traumatol Turc 2003;37:41–5 [in Turkish].

24. Naredo E, Cabero F, Beneyto P, et al. A randomized comparative study of short term response to blind injection versus sonographic-guided injection of local corticosteroids in patients with painful shoulder. J Rheumatol 2004;31:308–14.

25. Sofka CM, Collins AJ, Adler RS. Use of ultrasonographic guidance in interventional musculoskeletal procedures: a review from a single institution. J Ultrasound Med 2001;20:21–6.

26. Cardinal E, Chhem RK, Beauregard C. Ultrasound-guided interventional procedures in the musculoskeletal system. Radiol Clin North Am 1998;36: 597–604.

27. Bianchi S, Zamorani MP. US-guided interventional procedures. In: Baert AL, Knauth M, Sartor K, editors. Ultrasound of the musculoskeletal system. Berlin: Springer; 2006. p. 891–918.

28. Saucedo JM, Yaffe MA, Berschback JC, et al. Platelet-rich plasma. J Hand Surg Am 2012;37: 587–9.

29. McShane JM, Shah VN, Nazarian LN. Sonographically guided percutaneous needle tenotomy for treatment of common extensor tendinosis in the elbow: is a corticosteroid necessary? J Ultrasound Med 2008;27:1137–44.

30. Lohman M, Vasenius J, Nieminen O. Ultrasound guidance for puncture and injection in the radiocarpal joint. Acta Radiol 2007;48:744–7.

31. Grassi W, Lamanna G, Farina A, et al. Synovitis of small joints: sonographic guided diagnostic and therapeutic approach. Ann Rheum Dis 1999;58:595–7.

32. Umphrey GL, Brault JS, Hurdle MF, et al. Ultrasound-guided intra-articular injection of the trapeziometacarpal joint: description of technique. Arch Phys Med Rehabil 2008;89:153–6.

33. Grassi W, Farina A, Filippucci E, et al. Intralesional therapy in carpal tunnel syndrome: a sonographic-guided approach. Clin Exp Rheumatol 2002;20:73–6.

34. Qvistgaard E, Kristoffersen H, Terslev L, et al. Guidance by ultrasound of intra-articular injections in the knee and hip joints. Osteoarthritis Cartilage 2001;9: 512–7.

35. Rowbotham EL, Grainger AJ. Ultrasound-guided intervention around the hip joint. AJR Am J Roentgenol 2011;197:122–7.

36. Adler RS, Buly R, Ambrose R, et al. Diagnostic and therapeutic use of sonography-guided iliopsoas peritendinous injections. AJR Am J Roentgenol 2005;185:940–3.

37. Ryan M, Wong A, Rabago D, et al. Ultrasound-guided injections of hyperosmolar dextrose for overuse patellar tendinopathy: a pilot study. Br J Sports Med 2011;45:972–7.

38. Smith J, Finnoff JT, Santaella-Sante B, et al. Sonographically guided popliteus tendon sheath injection: techniques and accuracy. J Ultrasound Med 2010;29:775–82.

39. Sofka CM, Adler RS. Ultrasound-guided interventions in the foot and ankle. Semin Musculoskelet Radiol 2002;6:163–8.

40. Bruyn GA, Schmidt WA. How to perform ultrasound-guided injections. Best Pract Res Clin Rheumatol 2009;23:269–79.

Index

Note: Page numbers of article titles are in **boldface** type.

Ultrasound Clin 7 (2012) 551–556
http://dx.doi.org/10.1016/S1556-858X(12)00098-9
1556-858X/12/$ – see front matter © 2012 Elsevier Inc. All rights reserved.

ultrasound.theclinics.com

United States Postal Service

Statement of Ownership, Management, and Circulation
(All Periodicals Publications Except Requestor Publications)

1. Publication Title	2. Publication Number	3. Filing Date
Ultrasound Clinics	0 0 0 - 7 1 1	9/14/12

4. Issue Frequency	5. Number of Issues Published Annually	6. Annual Subscription Price
Jan/Apr/Jul/Oct	4	$243.00

7. Complete Mailing Address of Known Office of Publication (Not printer) (Street, city, county, state, and ZIP+4®)

Elsevier Inc.
360 Park Avenue South
New York, NY 10010-1710

Contact Person
Stephen Bushing
Telephone (Include area code)
215-239-3688

8. Complete Mailing Address of Headquarters or General Business Office of Publisher (Not printer)

Elsevier Inc., 360 Park Avenue South, New York, NY 10010-1710

9. Full Names and Complete Mailing Addresses of Publisher, Editor, and Managing Editor (Do not leave blank)
Publisher (Name and complete mailing address)

Kim Murphy, Elsevier, Inc., 1600 John F. Kennedy Blvd. Suite 1800, Philadelphia, PA 19103-2899
Editor (Name and complete mailing address)

Donald Mumford, Elsevier, Inc., 1600 John F. Kennedy Blvd. Suite 1800, Philadelphia, PA 19103-2899
Managing Editor (Name and complete mailing address)

Sarah Barth, Elsevier, Inc., 1600 John F. Kennedy Blvd. Suite 1800, Philadelphia, PA 19103-2899

10. Owner (Do not leave blank. If the publication is owned by a corporation, give the name and address of the corporation immediately followed by the names and addresses of all stockholders owning or holding 1 percent or more of the total amount of stock. If not owned by a corporation, give the names and addresses of the individual owners. If owned by a partnership or other unincorporated firm, give its name and address as well as those of each individual owner. If the publication is published by a nonprofit organization, give its name and address.)

Full Name	Complete Mailing Address
Wholly owned subsidiary of	1600 John F. Kennedy Blvd., Ste. 1800
Reed/Elsevier, US holdings	Philadelphia, PA 19103-2899

11. Known Bondholders, Mortgagees, and Other Security Holders Owning or Holding 1 Percent or More of Total Amount of Bonds, Mortgages, or Other Securities. If none, check box ☐ None

Full Name	Complete Mailing Address
N/A	

12. Tax Status (For completion by nonprofit organizations authorized to mail at nonprofit rates) (Check one)
The purpose, function, and nonprofit status of this organization and the exempt status for federal income tax purposes:
☐ Has Not Changed During Preceding 12 Months
☐ Has Changed During Preceding 12 Months (Publisher must submit explanation of change with this statement)

PS Form 3526, September 2007 (Page 1 of 3 (Instructions Page 3)) PSN 7530-01-000-9931 PRIVACY NOTICE: See our Privacy policy in www.usps.com

13. Publication Title	14. Issue Date for Circulation Data Below
Ultrasound Clinics	July 2012

15. Extent and Nature of Circulation		Average No. Copies Each Issue During Preceding 12 Months	No. Copies of Single Issue Published Nearest to Filing Date
a. Total Number of Copies (Net press run)		365	339
b. Paid Circulation (By Mail and Outside the Mail)	(1) Mailed Outside-County Paid Subscriptions Stated on PS Form 3541. (Include paid distribution above nominal rate, advertiser's proof copies, and exchange copies)	163	154
	(2) Mailed In-County Paid Subscriptions Stated on PS Form 3541 (Include paid distribution above nominal rate, advertiser's proof copies, and exchange copies)		
	(3) Paid Distribution Outside the Mails Including Sales Through Dealers and Carriers, Street Vendors, Counter Sales, and Other Paid Distribution Outside USPS®	37	48
	(4) Paid Distribution by Other Classes Mailed Through the USPS (e.g. First-Class Mail®)		
c. Total Paid Distribution (Sum of 15b (1), (2), (3), and (4))	▲	200	202
d. Free or Nominal Rate Distribution (By Mail and Outside the Mail)	(1) Free or Nominal Rate Outside-County Copies Included on PS Form 3541	45	52
	(2) Free or Nominal Rate In-County Copies Included on PS Form 3541		
	(3) Free or Nominal Rate Copies Mailed at Other Classes Through the USPS (e.g. First-Class Mail)		
	(4) Free or Nominal Rate Distribution Outside the Mail (Carriers or other means)		
e. Total Free or Nominal Rate Distribution (Sum of 15d (1), (2), (3) and (4)	▲	45	52
f. Total Distribution (Sum of 15c and 15e)	▲	245	254
g. Copies not Distributed (See instructions to publishers #4 (page #3))	▲	120	85
h. Total (Sum of 15f and g)	▲	365	339
i. Percent Paid (15c divided by 15f times 100)		81.63%	79.53%

16. Publication of Statement of Ownership
If the publication is a general publication, publication of this statement is required. Will be printed in the October 2012 issue of this publication. ☐ Publication not required

17. Signature and Title of Editor, Publisher, Business Manager, or Owner

[signature]
Stephen R. Bushing – Inventory/Distribution Coordinator

Date: September 14, 2012

I certify that all information furnished on this form is true and complete. I understand that anyone who furnishes false or misleading information on this form or who omits material or information requested on the form may be subject to criminal sanctions (including fines and imprisonment) and/or civil sanctions (including civil penalties).

PS Form 3526, September 2007 (Page 2 of 3)

Moving?

Make sure your subscription moves with you!

To notify us of your new address, find your **Clinics Account Number** (located on your mailing label above your name), and contact customer service at:

Email: journalscustomerservice-usa@elsevier.com

800-654-2452 (subscribers in the U.S. & Canada)
314-447-8871 (subscribers outside of the U.S. & Canada)

Fax number: 314-447-8029

Elsevier Health Sciences Division
Subscription Customer Service
3251 Riverport Lane
Maryland Heights, MO 63043

*To ensure uninterrupted delivery of your subscription, please notify us at least 4 weeks in advance of move.

Printed and bound by CPI Group (UK) Ltd, Croydon, CR0 4YY

03/10/2024

01040357-0004